Perinatal Mental Health

A Guide to the Edinburgh Postnatal Depression Scale (EPDS)

John Cox and Jeni Holden

To Karin

Gaskell is an imprint of the Royal College of Psychiatrists, 17 Belgrave Square, London SW1X 8PG, UK
http://www.rcpsych.ac.uk

British Library Cataloguing-in-Publication Data.
A catalogue record for this book is available from the British Library.
ISBN 1-901242-81-1

Distributed in North America by Balogh International Inc.

The Royal College of Psychiatrists is a registered charity (no. 228636).
Printed by Bell & Bain Limited, Glasgow, UK.

Contents

The authors

John Cox is a consultant psychiatrist and Emeritus Professor of Psychiatry at Keele University Medical School (Harplands Campus, Hilton Road, Harpfields, Stoke-on-Trent ST4 6TH, UK) and past-President of the Royal College of Psychiatrists.

Jeni Holden is retired psychology lecturer and former health visitor (c/o The Royal College of Psychiatrists, 17 Belgrave Square, London SW1X 8PG, UK)

Acknowledgements

The EPDS is used in many countries, and we thank all those who contributed much to its development, in particular, Ruth Sagovsky, who coauthored the first publication. Thanks also to the health visitors, doctors and midwives who helped with the research and made many useful suggestions, and especial thanks to the mothers and their partners who gave us permission to quote from interviews recorded during the counselling study.

We are grateful to our colleagues, in particular Sandra Elliott, Janice Gerrard and Carol Henshaw, who further developed the evidence base for using the EPDS in the community and provided many helpful comments on our manuscript, and to Richard Bambridge, who worked on the project and gave us his continuing support until his untimely death.

Preface

The Edinburgh Postnatal Depression Scale (EPDS) is a 10-item self-report scale devised as a screening questionnaire to improve the detection of postnatal depression in the community. This book is written to provide readers in different countries with updated and accessible information on the scale and its use in primary and secondary care. Appendix 1 includes the original scale and a score sheet, and Appendix 2 shows some of the foreign-language versions.

Depressive disorders are one of the most common causes of disability worldwide. According to the 1999 World Health Report (World Health Organization, 1999), unipolar major depression accounts for 4.2% of the world's total burden of disease as measured by 'disability adjusted life years' (DALYS) and is the fifth leading cause of disability.

Postnatal depression, which affects women at a time of maximum vulnerability and can last untreated for many years, is one of the main contributors to this disconcerting statistic. Yet, as we show in this text, the possibility of secondary prevention through early identification is consistent with the evidence base and is being actively considered by national governments in many countries, led by primary care professionals.

The EPDS was developed in the 1980s because clinical experience in both rich and poor countries showed that unipolar depression, and postnatal depression in particular, is a common disorder that causes much unnecessary misery for women and their families. We were also becoming aware that such depression can adversely affect the development and nutrition of the infant, the continuity of the marriage and the economy of the household.

Since then, worldwide communications have become almost instantaneous, women's health issues have developed a higher profile and the knowledge base of perinatal mental health and perinatal psychiatry has increased substantially. The Marcé Society (an interdisciplinary society that stimulates research and provides a forum for disseminating information about perinatal mental health) has flourished and become more truly international; the voices of women are now more clearly heard, as qualitative research methods complement a quantitative approach; voluntary patient and carer groups are influencing governments and changing mental health priorities.

Within this context the EPDS has provided a timely stimulus to considering the prevention of postnatal depression. In the UK, primary care professionals are now more skilled in detecting such depression and providing a range of evidence-based therapies. The EPDS has also facilitated much epidemiological research by its use as a first-stage screening measure. Furthermore, because of its sensitivity to change over time, it can be used as an outcome measure in treatment studies.

Although the scale was devised to meet the needs of quantitative research as well as for clinical use, it has opened up an important qualitative debate about the meaning of symptoms, the equivalence of metaphor (e.g. 'things have been getting on top of me') and the cross-cultural validity of a scale developed from within a specific social context.

It is remarkable that the UK debate about the use and misuse of the EPDS should have moved on from a local consideration to a matter for a National Screening Committee, which has rightly pointed out deficiencies in the evidence base that must be addressed before national universal screening can be put firmly in place.

The response of the Community Practitioners' and Health Visitors' Association (CPHVA) has been equally committed. Health visitors, only too familiar with the consequences of untreated perinatal mental disorder, have already taken the lead role in screening for this common and treatable disorder. They have become familiar with the skills and consequences of conducting clinical assessment interviews and, in particular, recognise the usefulness of the EPDS when administered by a fully trained health professional. The EPDS does not screen for those at risk of becoming depressed in the future but it will identify a mild depression, which can rapidly develop into a severe, prolonged disorder.

The evidence base for the optimum use of the EPDS must continue to be explored. We hope that its wider use will facilitate long-overdue treatment trials. Above all we hope that the EPDS will continue to encourage practitioners to listen to women, to take what they say and how they say it seriously, and also to collect data that will lead to a higher priority being given to perinatal mental health and women's health issues in general.

The training of obstetricians, general practitioners, midwives, health visitors, psychiatrists and psychologists is still deficient in many aspects of psychosomatic obstetrics and perinatal care. We hope that this handbook will help to change things, increasing the chances for new mothers to establish a good relationship with their infants and an optimal environment in which the children may develop.

We hope that our book will encourage researchers and clinicians across the world to develop perinatal mental health strategies and to search for ways of preventing a condition that can reduce the quality of life for the parents – and for the next generation.

CHAPTER 1

Postnatal depression: an overview

'My husband wants another baby. The idea is quite nice, but it really frightens me to think that after having the baby I would be like this again. I wouldn't mind the morning sickness or the actual birth. It is the postnatal depression that really frightens me. I don't think I could face that again. It was horrific.' (Holden, 1988)

Introduction

Postnatal depression affects not only the quality of a woman's own life and her experience of mothering but also her infant, her other children, her partner and everyone around her, including those involved in her care. On an individual level, the experience can be devastating. Pitt (1968) noted that many of the women in his early study felt quite changed from their normal self, and most 'had never been depressed like this before'. Without help or treatment, the consequences may be long term and expensive for the women, for their families and in the demands made on health care resources. In severe depression, especially with psychotic symptoms, there is a risk of suicide. This is shown in *The Confidential Enquiries into Maternal Deaths in the United Kingdom* (Oates, 2001), which record that psychological causes were the most common cause of maternal deaths in the triennium 1996–1999.

The term 'postnatal depression' is commonly used to describe a sustained depressive disorder in women following childbirth; the condition is characterised by a low, sad mood, lack of interest, anxiety, sleep difficulties, reduced self-esteem, somatic symptoms such as headache and weight loss, and difficulty coping with day-to-day tasks. The term was used by Vivienne Welburn (1980) in the title of a popular book and by Ann Oakley (1980) to describe a sustained depressive disorder occurring in women in the first year after childbirth. It was also used in the Edinburgh study (Cox *et al*, 1982) to describe women experiencing depression within 3 months of childbirth. Cox *et al* offer the conservative estimate of 13% for the prevalence of depression at that time and report that half of these women were not identified by the local primary care service. In the USA, the term 'post-partum depression' is more commonly used to describe mothers with a non-psychotic mood disorder (for a review of the US literature see O'Hara, 1995).

Participants at a workshop in Sweden (organised by Birgitta Wickberg, Philip Hwang and J.C.) concluded that the term 'postnatal depression' is useful to describe any depressive disorder without psychotic features present within the first year following childbirth; the limitation of the 4-week specifier in DSM–IV (American Psychiatric Association, 1994) and 6 weeks in ICD–10 (World Health Organization, 1992) was recognised.

In the late 1970s and throughout the 1980s postnatal depression was largely considered to be a Western phenomenon, with infrequent documentation in the cross-cultural literature. This suggested that it might be a 'culture-bound' phenomenon. Possible contributing factors were thought to be the lack of social structuring of the event of childbirth, combined with a lack of accompanying ritual and support for the mother (Stern & Kruckman, 1983; Cox, 1996). Research over the past 10 years, however, has increasingly revealed that depression is a negative outcome of childbirth for women in diverse countries and cultures.

The public health importance of postnatal depression is now more widely acknowledged in mental health policy guidance both in the UK and in other countries than formerly because of the suffering and disability of the woman and the disruption of the family at a time of maximum vulnerability. The evidence of depression having an adverse effect on the mother–infant relationship and on child development is also more widely recognised.

It is well established that postnatal depression affects at least 10% of women within the first post-partum year and that even higher rates occur in urban areas of deprivation. Cooper *et al* (1999), for example, found that a third of women in an African township in Capetown had a serious major depressive disorder. Similarly, Cryan *et al* (2001) found 28.6% of 944 women in a socially deprived urban area in Dublin, Ireland, had depression postnatally. The frequency of depression is much lower in cohesive island communities such as Malta (Felice, 1998) or in affluent societies with generous maternity benefits such as Sweden (Wickberg & Hwang, 1997). It is also less common in cultures with more clearly defined parental roles such as Japan (Tamaki *et al*, 1997) and Malaysia (the majority of Malaysian women still retain traditional postnatal beliefs and practices (Kit *et al*, 1997)) and in countries where childbirth gives high status to the married mother (Cox, 1983).

Postnatal depression is not, however, a specific discrete disorder fundamentally different from depression occurring at other times, and our use of the term does not indicate that such depression always develops after delivery or is necessarily caused by the specific stress of childbirth. Pitt (1968) considered depression after childbirth to be 'atypical', although we ourselves did not find the symptoms different from depression at other times, for example in mothers with older children (Cox *et al*, 1996). Nor was there evidence in a Stoke-on-Trent study (Murray *et al*, 1995) that the range of depressive symptoms distinguished between early-onset (i.e. within the first 6 weeks) and later-onset depression. A study by Henshaw (2000) has confirmed, however, that severe 'postnatal blues' (see below) is a powerful predictor of a subsequent depression: 40% of women with severe postnatal blues subsequently developed a depressive disorder. These findings suggest that the birth event can be an important neuroendocrine trigger for a more sustained depressive disorder. Cooper & Murray (1995) studied two groups of primiparous women for 5 years and found that women for whom the index postnatal episode was a recurrence of depression were at raised risk of further non-post-partum episodes but not of post-partum episodes. Women for whom the index postnatal episode was the first experience of depression were at raised risk for further episodes of postnatal depression but not for non-post-partum episodes. They concluded that their findings supported the use of postnatal depression as a specific diagnostic entity.

Although in perhaps 15% of cases, postnatal depression has an antenatal onset, Brugha *et al* (1998, 2000) found that both antenatal prediction and prevention of postnatal depression seem to be totally unsuccessful. In their prospective cohort study, 507 women were interviewed during pregnancy and followed up at 3 months post-partum. In a randomised controlled trial, 190 pregnant women were then randomly assigned to a structured intervention or to a control group. There were no significant differences between the groups on either postnatal depression or risk factors. The authors claim that 'predictors of depressive symptoms development differ from predictors of recovery from clinical depression in women' (Brugha *et al*, 1998: p. 63). It seems likely, therefore, that there are powerful causal factors specific to the immediate postnatal weeks.

Other postnatal psychiatric disorders

Postnatal depression is generally distinguished from puerperal psychosis by its later onset following childbirth (4–6 weeks) and by the absence of florid delusions, hallucinations and gross behavioural disturbance that can characterise a puerperal psychosis. Research findings suggest that the puerperal psychoses are linked in their aetiology and prognosis to the bipolar mood disorders ('manic–depression') and that they have a strong tendency to recur following subsequent pregnancies (a risk of at least 1 in 4) (Kendell *et al*, 1981; Wieck *et al*, 1991). Although rare (2 per 1000 deliveries), the puerperal psychoses can have devastating consequences for the mother (suicide) and the infant (infanticide) (Kendell *et al*, 1987; Marks & Kumar, 1993). Their optimal management usually requires the full resources of a perinatal mental health team with access to a purpose-built mother and baby unit, as recommended by the Royal College of Psychiatrists (2000). With comprehensive treatment, however, the prognosis is usually good, although there is a high risk of recurrence. Women affected should therefore be closely monitored in all subsequent pregnancies and after delivery, when appropriate prevention strategies should be in place, provided by specialist perinatal mental health teams.

'Postnatal blues' describes the transitory mood disturbances (emotional lability and crying) found in at least two-thirds of women in the first week post-partum and particularly on day 5 (Cox *et al*, 1982). An understanding of postnatal blues is important for a number of reasons, including the following:

- they are distressing and perplexing for the mother and her family, and there is therefore a need for an explanation of their causes and for support and reassurance;
- severe blues can be difficult to distinguish from the premonitory signs of a puerperal psychosis and from the early onset of a non-psychotic postnatal depression;
- increased understanding of the neuroendocrine causes of post-natal blues will contribute to knowledge about the effect of sex steroids on central neurotransmitter systems and provide a window for further understanding of postnatal mood disorder.

The relationship between postnatal disorders is shown in Fig. 1.1, which illustrates the maintaining factors ('vicious circles') of postnatal depression and how the lack of culturally sanctioned family support can both cause and be a consequence of a prolonged depressive disorder at this time.

Other important psychiatric disorders found in the puerperium include panic disorder, obsessive–compulsive disorder, post-traumatic

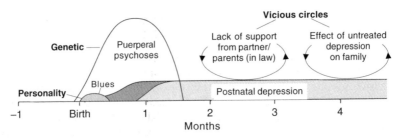

Fig. 1.1 Causal and maintaining factors of postnatal depression (after Cox, 1998).

stress disorder and generalised anxiety disorder. Women with these disorders may score highly on the Edinburgh Postnatal Depression Scale (EPDS; Cox *et al*, 1987), especially if they have a depressed mood, which is a common accompaniment of these conditions. The EPDS, however, may not detect the less-common disorders listed above, or a severe mental illness such as schizophrenia, or alcoholism, substance misuse or an organic confusional state.

Women's narratives

Mothers themselves often describe their depression and its effects quite graphically. In tape-recorded interviews conducted after a randomised controlled trial of counselling by health visitors (Holden, 1988) women expressed their feelings in the following way:

'I have never felt like that in my life before. Nobody could speak to me because I would burst into tears at the least thing. I took an extreme dislike to everybody in this world except my baby. I wanted everybody to go away, I was interested in nothing.'

'It was terrible. It was like someone else taking over. I wasn't the same person any more. I didn't recognise myself. It wasn't me, that was what I kept saying. It wasn't me.'

'It was absolutely ghastly. It felt as if there was a physical weight inside that was dragging me down. I was pulling it around all the time; everything was an effort.'

Another mother told us that something had 'got a hold of her' which she knew was serious and required medical help. We found that for at least a half of the women who became depressed the disorder lasted for a year and sometimes merged into a second postnatal depression that followed a subsequent pregnancy (Cox *et al*, 1984). Many women clearly recalled postnatal depression several years later.

Effects on interactions with infants

Postnatal depression occurs when heavy demands are placed on women's resources and when infant learning and development are taking place:

'Mothers of young infants, especially when it is their first child, must adjust to their baby and learn to understand the infant's communications and needs. This task is more difficult if the mothers are feeling despondent, fatigued and overwhelmed by the responsibilities attendant upon transition to parenthood ... [T]he sadness, irritability and social withdrawal that characterise depressed women compromise their ability to provide a sensitive, nurturing environment for their babies.' (Campbell & Cohn, 1997: p. 166)

After completing our counselling intervention study many woman told us of the effect that depression had had on their relationship with their infant. One woman had seriously feared harming her baby, and constantly fantasised while bathing him about how easy it would be to push his head under the water. Others said:

'It was lonely and I felt as if I was inside this box, just all by myself, with nobody to talk to and nobody to help me. I started taking my anger out on [my baby]. I never hit him, but I grabbed him. Or I used to ignore him, let him scream, shut him away. I wasn't loving him like a mother should.'

'It really bothered me to be depressed when I had such a lovely baby, it didn't seem fair to her. I never stopped loving her, but I couldn't express it. I was withdrawn into myself. I liked the baby but I wasn't interested in her. I just did things automatically and I wouldn't remember doing them. It was as if I wasn't really there. I felt I was a failure as a mother.' (Holden, 1988)

One health visitor became concerned that another mother showed little interest in her baby, leaving him entirely to her sister to look after. This woman told me that she had felt she was not a good enough mother, and that the baby would know this and reject her.

The accounts cited above are retrospective (between 9 and 12 months post-partum), describing how the women had felt in the early months. As the depression resolved, they were able to engage with their babies in a more caring and loving manner.

Adverse effects on the mother–infant relationship and the feelings of both mother and baby are well documented. Murray *et al* (1996a) found, in a comparison with well women, that at 2 months post-partum mothers with depression were less sensitively attuned to their infants and were less affirming and more negating of infant experience. Murray *et al* suggested that persistent patterns of withdrawn behaviour may in this way be set up in the baby which could limit subsequent experience and development, even after the mother has recovered and is responding more affectionately.

Research groups are now looking increasingly closely at the ways in which these mother–infant interactions are disturbed. A preliminary study by Kaplan *et al* (1999) of the long-term impact of postnatal depressed mood on mother–child interaction demonstrated for the first time that 4-month-old babies react with far less interest to the speech of mothers with depression. The tape-recorded voices of non-depressed mothers were more likely to stimulate their infants' interest and the time they spent focusing on an abstract pattern. Edhborg *et al* (2001) suggested that the young children of women with high EPDS scores develop 'representations' of their mother and of their interactions with her as being less joyful than do the children of mothers without depression, and that these representations may remain beyond the period of the mother's depressed mood.

Persistence of effects on children of mothers with depression

There is considerable evidence of a sustained adverse affect of maternal depression on later cognitive development (Wrate et al, 1985; Cogill et al, 1986; Cox, 1988; Murray, 1988; Stein et al, 1991; Murray et al, 1996b). Disturbances in early mother–infant interactions were found to be predictive of poorer infant cognitive outcome at 18 months of age (Cooper & Murray, 1997). In children 3½ years of age and at school entry both postnatal and more recent maternal depression were associated with significantly raised levels of child disturbance, particularly among boys and those from lower social class families (Sharp et al, 1995; Sinclair & Murray, 1998). These unwanted effects may persist even longer. In a study of long-term sequelae in the children of mothers who were depressed at 3 months post-partum, for example, Hay et al (2001) found that 11-year-old children, especially boys, had significantly lower IQ scores, more attentional and reading problems, greater difficulties in mathematical reasoning and were more likely to have special educational needs than children of mothers who had not had post-partum depression. There is some evidence, however, that such effects can be changed by an intervention to help the mother during depression (see Chapter 5).

Fathers and postnatal depression

Postnatal depression in the mother commonly has a profound effect on her partner and on their relationship. Fathers may themselves become depressed. In Birmingham, UK, Ballard et al (1994) studied 200 couples post-partum and found that the prevalence of depression (ascertained by the earlier 13-item EPDS) in fathers was 9.0% at 6 weeks after the birth and 5.4% at 6 months. As expected, mothers had a significantly higher prevalence of caseness at both 6 weeks and 6 months post-partum than fathers had, but fathers were significantly more likely to be cases if their partners had depression. In a longitudinal study in Portugal, Areias et al (1996a) found that in the first 3 months post-partum, nearly a quarter of the women shown to be at risk in pregnancy became depressed, in contrast with less than 5% of their partners. In the next 9 months, however, men were more prone to becoming depressed than previously and their depressions tended to follow the earlier onset of depression in their partner.

Matthey et al (2001), who validated the EPDS for use with fathers, found a relatively low level of depression in men compared with the level for their postnatal partners. However, distress was more likely in the father when the mother was also distressed.

After our counselling study, the fathers were asked about their experiences during their partners' depression:

'It was terrible. No matter what you do you are wrong. She was awfully quick tempered; things she would normally laugh about just make her mad. She had changed a lot. Before, if we had a lovers' tiff, in the finish we would start laughing at how stupid we were. But now, the least little thing and she starts to cry. I've been kicked out of the house hundreds of times, but I never went. I could see there was something wrong with her, and she was telling me it was the depression, but I used to say to myself "is this just an excuse she is using, is she really tired of me, does she really want me to go?"' (Holden, 1988)

Although in this study we had not set out to look at depression in fathers, several of the partners of women in the study themselves spoke of feeling depressed, and it was clear that the wife's depression caused considerable disruption to the relationship of the majority of couples. In tape-recorded interviews, both men and women spoke of a loss of affectionate closeness:

'If he puts his arms around me I absolutely shudder. I say "Oh, Dave don't come near me!" And it is pretty frightening because I have never been that way. All the time that I've known Dave we used to sit and cuddle each other, we were always very close, but now he sits over there and I sit over here.' (Holden, 1988)

Many couples who had been in the group that received counselling reported that this support had sustained or even improved their relationship. Without help, however, depression can lead to relationship breakdown. In the control group, one husband left his wife completely because he could not cope with the unpredictability of her moods. Another left for 3 months but came back after his wife had recovered from her depression. Almost a year after his first baby was born, another husband said that he had often thought of leaving:

'It was great before the baby came. But now ... I'd be as well being a monk. What matters in a marriage, well, it's nine-tenths of a marriage, is sex and, well ... and love. And if you can't get even a cuddle, nobody's going to stay around.' (Holden, 1988)

Couples told us that they were totally unprepared for the possibility of depression and claimed that it had not been explained or even mentioned in antenatal preparation classes. It is hoped that the increasing awareness of health professionals will improve both prenatal and postnatal information given to new parents.

Clinical perspectives

The presentation of postnatal depression was usefully summarised by Brice Pitt (1968) in his pioneer study of London women. He emphasised the way in which depressive symptoms were often coloured by the mother's relationship with her baby and the need to understand additional stressors caused by mothering. Pitt described postnatal depression as follows:

'[The women experience] tearfulness, despondency, feelings of inadequacy and inability to cope – particularly with the baby ... Guilt was mainly confined to self-reproach over not loving or caring enough for the baby ... Many felt quite changed from their usual selves, and most had never been depressed like this before.

'Depression was almost invariably accompanied, and sometimes over-shadowed, by ... anxiety over the baby [which] was not justified by the babies' health ...

'Unusual irritability was common, sometimes adding to feelings of guilt. A few patients complained of impaired concentration and memory. Undue fatigue and ready exhaustion were frequent, so that mothers could barely deal with their babies, let alone look after the rest of the family and cope with housework and shopping.

'Anorexia ... was present with remarkable consistence. Sleep disturbance, over and above that inevitable with a new baby, was reported by a third of the patients.'

Identifying postnatal depression

This present book describes the way in which the EPDS can improve the detection of postnatal depression in the community, sometimes as an additional component of a clinical interview. In an earlier publication (Cox, 1989) it was suggested that one or all of the following could alert the obstetrician, midwife, health visitor or general practitioner that a mother has depression:

- a complaint of feeling low, worried, fatigued or having severe sleep difficulties;
- constant complaints of somatic symptoms such as headaches, abdominal pain or breast tenderness, without an adequate physical cause;
- an expressed fear that the doctor or health visitor will be excessively critical of her mothering ability, and may even be considering taking away her baby;
- excessive concern about the baby's health and preoccupation with minimal feeding difficulties; continuous over-solicitousness and immediate response to the baby's demands;
- unexpected failure to attend a postnatal clinic or child health clinic;
- a baby who is failing to thrive and crying excessively.

Michael O'Hara has described the clinical presentation in the USA in the following way:

'About day 3 post-partum, Mrs Jones's mood began to sink. She said that her low mood felt almost like physical pain. She also reported feeling anxious and irritable at this time. During the period of her depression, which lasted at least 2 months, she completely lost her appetite. She woke up during the night and could not get back to sleep. She commented that it was almost like not falling asleep. She had no energy and lost interest in most things. Mrs Jones reported feeling guilty; in particular, she believed that she wasn't a good mother, and she blamed herself for her son's colic. She also had extreme difficulty in concentrating. Finally, she found that her work and family relationships were "impaired by her depression". Despite both her mother and husband urging her to seek help for her depression, she did not. At 6 months post-partum, she was still reporting a moderate level of depressive symptomatology.' (O'Hara, 1995: p. 9).

Confirmation of the diagnosis

If a mother is assessed by a health worker as being 'possibly depressed' or has a high score on the EPDS, then specific enquiry should be made about the presence or absence of the following depressive symptoms or complaints:

- *Depressed mood* Most women recognise when they are down, sad, depressed, low-spirited or 'blue'. Asking the question 'How do you feel in your spirits these days?' will usually elicit this crucial information. The health professional can then determine the extent to which this depressed mood is a break from the usual mood state, and establish how long the mood has lasted and how distressed the mother is. A depressed mood which has lasted for at least 4 weeks and is accompanied by other symptoms of depression would strongly suggest that the mother has clinical depression.
- *Excessive anxiety* Although being anxious (fearful, worried) can occur in the absence of a depressed mood, if anxiety *is* present it should be regarded as coexisting with depression unless shown not to be so. It is wise to assume that any mother who is anxious is also likely to be depressed.
- *Lack of interest and pleasure in doing things* Anhedonia is a hallmark of depression. The lack of interest may show itself through an unusual disinterest in cooking, reading or in resuming sexual relations – libido is often non-existent.
- *Early morning wakening* Early morning wakening when not caused by a noisy baby or a restless partner is characteristic of depression; when consistently present and prolonged it is especially typical of the depressed phase of a bipolar disorder. Initial insomnia, when the

mother is kept awake by rounds of worrying thoughts or by an exaggerated need to listen to any sound from her baby, may be another sign of a depressive illness.

• *Ideas of not coping, self-blame and guilt.*

The clinical skills required to determine the presence or absence of these symptoms of depressive disorder can usually be acquired during supervised undergraduate or postgraduate training or from a post-qualifying refresher course for primary care health professionals.

Women with depression who have fixed delusional ideas of guilt or self-blame congruent with their depressed mood are best described as having severe depression. It is very important to identify this group of women in primary care because they may have increased risk of self-harm and may require treatment with antidepressants and *immediate* referral to a specialist team.

The ICD–10 primary care criteria for a depressive disorder [F32] can be recommended for use by general practitioners. These criteria specifically identify women who have given birth as being at high risk.

Causes

The possible causes of postnatal depression can usually be ascertained only after a full clinical history has been obtained from the mother and her family. A biopsychosocial approach should be used when establishing causes, and this includes understanding the way that the social environment may influence the expression of genes and the likelihood of adverse life events. The causal domains involved are illustrated in Fig. 1.2.

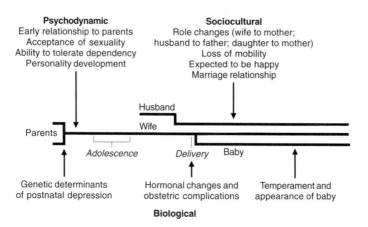

Fig. 1.2   Possible causal factors in postnatal depression (after Cox, 1986: p. 39).

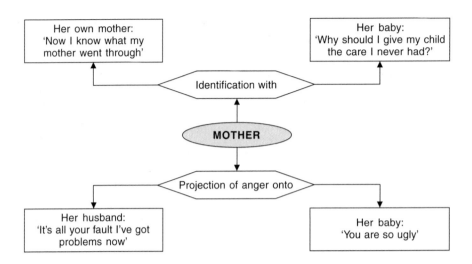

Fig. 1.3 Identification and projection: common psychological defence mechanisms in the puerperium (after Cox, 1986: p. 35).

Present preoccupations of society with postnatal depression and the popularity of the label may reflect a greater concern about women's health issues in general, the status of childbearing in society and the increased vulnerability of modern families. In almost all societies depression can be identified post-partum, but the *meaning* of this condition for the mother and her family will vary. Local popular explanations may include biological (hormonal), social (lack of support) and psychological factors (e.g. 'my baby is making me depressed') (Fig. 1.3).

In the developing world or in societies riven by warfare a mother's inability to obtain basic essentials (food, clothes and warmth) for herself or her children may provoke additional hardship, exclusion, hopelessness and eventually clinical depression.

There is no simple single cause for postnatal depression: a review of the literature will provide a list of variables associated with depression, each of which may or may not be specifically causal. Findings from our own studies suggest that the following are associated with postnatal depression in mothers: the previous personality of the mother (always being a 'worrier'); a previous history of mental disorder; earlier loss of the mother's own mother; severe postnatal blues; giving up work reluctantly; and a poor relationship with the mother's mother (see also Holden, 1991).

There is now greater understanding of the way that oestrogen receptors influence central neurotransmitter systems. Recent genetic studies (Coyle *et al*, 2000) have found an increase in the 12 allele of the serotonin (5-HT) transporter gene in women with a susceptibility to bipolar disorder who develop puerperal psychosis. Researchers are now searching for the puerperal trigger of puerperal psychosis.

Future studies of brain function might show the way in which a crying baby, fractious husband or intrusive mother-in-law could modify brain functions in the post-partum period, and how these difficulties in a susceptible mother might provoke mental disorder. The evidence for such a specific neurobiological trigger for post-partum mood disorder is at present circumstantial, but the finding (Henshaw, 2000) that women with severe blues have a one in four risk of developing a subsequent major depression is a strong pointer to pursuing this line of research enquiry.

However, the results of the International Transcultural Study of Postnatal Depression show that when women themselves are asked to describe the cause of unhappiness before and after childbirth they give explanations almost entirely in the social domain (see Oates *et al*, 2003). Indeed, it is popularly assumed that the primary cause of postnatal mood disorder is the meaning that women attach to events and to the lack of instrumental and psychological support; interestingly only rarely do women attribute postnatal mood disturbances to a disorder of brain function caused by hormonal changes.

It is nevertheless possible that physiological changes in the mother in the immediate post-partum months do increase the likelihood of emotional disturbances, but that the emotions experienced are contingent on the memories laid down in earlier formative relationships, on the nature and availability of social support and, in particular, on the meaning for the mother of giving birth to a dependent infant.

Caring for women with postnatal depression

The main use of the EPDS in routine clinical work is to assist in the secondary prevention of postnatal depression by identifying this disorder as early as possible so that therapy can be initiated. Supportive counselling by a primary care worker such as a health visitor, midwife or practice nurse can be particularly effective for women with a mild disorder (Holden *et al*, 1989). Assistance from a mental health worker with a special interest in perinatal mental disorder is necessary for women who remain depressed despite counselling, for those at risk of suicide and in situations in which the baby is at risk of neglect or physical abuse by the mother. Women who have developed a depressive disorder with psychotic features (delusions of guilt, self-blame or persecution) will also need care from a specialist perinatal team. If other members of the family also have mental health problems or the stress has affected older children, then the skills of a family-oriented psychiatric team are very important. In this context, the use of the Care Programme Approach and the development of a care plan to coordinate multi-professional working that includes the mother and her family are useful. For women with severe mental disorder or those recovering from a psychosis multi-professional management strategies, including child protection and the identification of a keyworker, are recommended.

The present book does not describe in detail the treatment options for women with severe postnatal depression who require specialist help from secondary services. Other sources (e.g. Oates, 1989; Brockington, 1996; Stein, 1998) must therefore be consulted for this information. The principles of the treatment approach, however, do not differ substantially from the treatment of depression at other times, although the social context of new parenting, the presence of a dependent infant and the specific features of a risk assessment in the puerperium need always to be considered.

In Chapter 5 we give particular emphasis to the benefit of counselling by primary care workers. It is important to stress, however, that this approach alone is likely to benefit only women with mild to moderate depression and that the combination of counselling with antidepressant medication is necessary for women with severe depression.

CHAPTER 2

The origins and development of the Edinburgh Postnatal Depression Scale

The development of the Edinburgh Postnatal Depression Scale (EPDS) was first described by Cox et al in 1987 and was subsequently summarised in *Perinatal Psychiatry* (Cox & Holden, 1994). In these publications we suggested that the EPDS would help in identifying postnatal depressive disorders which would otherwise be undetected in the community. Prospective studies of postnatal depression in Uganda and Scotland had found frequencies of 10% and 13% respectively (Cox, 1983). These were striking findings which at the time increased awareness of the need to develop methods to detect this disabling mood disorder. Depression in the African mothers living in villages north of Kampala prevented them from working (digging and carrying water) and most received no help at all from traditional healers or health professionals. The Scottish women also struggled to meet the demands of their baby and their partner.

Existing scales

It was apparent that existing self-report scales for depression were unlikely to be useful in detecting depression in childbearing women. The State of Anxiety and Depression (SAD) self-report scale of Bedford & Foulds (1978), the Beck Depression Inventory (BDI; Beck et al, 1961) and the General Health Questionnaire (GHQ; Goldberg, 1972) all had serious limitations for use with pregnant and post-partum women. Women might endorse (tick) the somatic items on the scales because of the physiological changes of childbearing (e.g. weight gain, breathlessness and tachycardia), and childbearing women can disclose normal worries. Sleep difficulty as a symptom of depression is difficult to evaluate when sleep is being disturbed by the baby.

In 1983 we noted that such 'false positives' in self-report questionnaires might reduce the reliable detection of neurosis in pregant and post-partum women, and that scales specifically for use during pregnancy and in the puerperium might be needed (Cox, 1983). Snaith (1983), who had developed the Hospital Anxiety and Depression (HAD) scale (Zigmond & Snaith, 1983), also recognised the need to modify existing self-report scales for use in specific clinical situations. Williams *et al*

(1980) had emphasised that questionnaires validated for use on hospital samples should be revalidated when used in the community. Thus, by the mid-1980s the need to develop a depression scale specifically validated for use by childbearing women was apparent and increasingly compelling.

Validating the Edinburgh Postnatal Depression Scale

At the outset we recognised that a questionnaire for use with child-bearing women would need to be simple to complete and acceptable to people who did not regard themselves as unwell. Furthermore, the healthcare worker administering the scale might not have had any specialised training in psychiatric disorders. Finally, the new scale would need to have satisfactory validity and reliability, and be sensitive to changes in the severity of depression over time.

Clinical experience when assessing and treating women with postnatal depression was used to identify possible items from question-naires such as the SAD and HAD scales and the BDI. Items that lacked 'face validity' (i.e. that would not have been understood by childbearing women or might have been inappropriate at this time, e.g. 'I can enjoy a good book or radio or television' or 'I feel as if I am slowed down') and 'somatic' items (misleading as indicators of depression) were discarded. We then selected 30 items, which included several of our own construction, to pilot with women who were asked to comment about the wording and the order of the items.

We eventually agreed on 13 items that we thought likely to detect mothers with clinical depression. The resultant questionnaire was then validated (Cox, 1986) on a sample of 60 postnatal women, who completed the 13-item scale and were interviewed by the psychiatrist Ruth Sagovsky using Goldberg et al's (1970) Clinical Interview Schedule. The diagnosis of depression using major and minor Research Diagnostic Criteria (RDC; Spitzer et al, 1978) was then established. The 13-item scale was found to distinguish satisfactorily between women with and without depression. A factor analysis, however, showed not only a 'depression' factor that explained 46% of the variance but also another factor that loaded on three items ('I have enjoyed being a mother' and the two irritability items). We therefore realised that the 13-item scale could be shortened to 10 without impairing its effectiveness. This shortened 10-item scale (named the Edinburgh Postnatal Depression Scale) had no specific item about mothering the baby nor about irritability, a development that later widened the potential use of the scale to other populations.

A second validation of the 10-item version was carried out on a sample of 84 postnatal women who were taking part in an ongoing

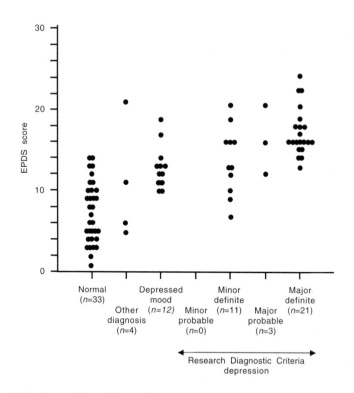

Fig. 2.1 Validation of the 10-item Edinburgh Postnatal Depression Scale (EPDS; Cox *et al*, 1987).

study of health visitor counselling (Fig. 2.1) (Cox *et al*, 1987). The shortened scale identified all women with a definite major depression and two of the three with a probable major depression at a cut-off of 12/13. Of the 11 women with a definite minor depression, only four had a false-negative score. Although this cut-off resulted in 11 false positives, 6 of these women had several depressive symptoms without fulfilling all RDC for clinical depression. Interestingly, three women with a psychiatric diagnosis other than depression all scored below the cut-off.

The sensitivity of the EPDS (the proportion of women with RDC depression who were true positives) was 86%, and the specificity (proportion of RDC non-depressed women who were true negatives) was 78%. The positive predictive value (the proportion of women above the threshold on the EPDS ($n = 41$) who met RDC for depression ($n = 30$)) was 73%. These findings suggested that the rate for failing to detect women with depression could be reduced to under 10% by using a lower cut-off, of 9/10. This was the cut-off that we recommended in our initial publication of the EPDS for use as a first-stage screening measure.

Reliability

The split-half reliability of the 10-item EPDS was 0.88 and the standardised α coefficient 0.87. (The split-half reliability was obtained by dividing items on the scale into two halves, which were then compared; a high correlation suggested that the items were measuring the same characteristics.) The sensitivity to change in severity of depression over time was established by comparing EPDS scores obtained at two interviews separated by a 3-month interval. This showed that the EPDS can be used to detect changes in the level of depression over time, so widening its use as an outcome measure in intervention studies.

The three women with a false-negative score each had other family members present when they were interviewed. We recommend that the EPDS is optimally completed when other family members are not present, as women may exaggerate or minimise their problems in these circumstances. The 10-item EPDS was found to be very acceptable to most of the women and, as important, to their health visitors. Another advantage of the scale was its brevity and simplicity of scoring.

These findings, together with our clinical experience, suggested that the EPDS would be useful in detecting postnatal depression in the community as well as in research projects. A cut-off of 9/10 was likely to detect almost all cases of depression, with very few false negatives. This cut-off score is particularly useful in a research project in which the EPDS is the only measure used or when it is used as a first-stage screening scale to identify possible depression. Another advantage of the EPDS in epidemiological studies is that it can elicit a high response rate (95–97%) when sent by post, especially if there had been previous contact with the research team and there is follow-up of women who do not initially respond (Murray & Carothers, 1990; Roy et al, 1993).

In the community, the EPDS is useful in the secondary prevention of postnatal depression by identifying the early onset of depressive symptoms. It can be administered by a trained health visitor, practice nurse or midwife at a postnatal or child health clinic or on a home visit. When using the EPDS in primary care settings as a component of a screening programme, the 9/10 cut-off may be over-inclusive, so a cut-off of 12/13 is often recommended. It should be remembered that the EPDS screens only for depression and also that women who score below the cut-off may none the less have depression.

The scale is best administered by a health professional who is familiar with mental health problems and has had training in their evidence base. A woman with a high score or an unexpectedly low score should be further assessed by a health professional and/or referred to a general practitioner, mental health nurse, psychologist or psychiatrist. A mother with profound depression might not grasp the meaning of the items; others may wish to cover up their disability or fear stigma or the shame of not coping.

Comparison with other scales

Several studies have compared the performance of the EPDS and other depression questionnaires for use in the postnatal period.

In the UK (Wales), Harris et al (1989) compared the EPDS and the BDI in their abilities to identify subjects who had major depression according to DSM–III criteria (American Psychiatric Association, 1980). The sensitivity of the EPDS was 95% and its specificity 93%. They concluded that the performance of the BDI was markedly inferior in this application, with a sensitivity of 68% and specificity of 88%.

In a Canadian study, Lussier et al (1996) found a low concordance between the BDI and the EPDS. Their analysis revealed distinct response patterns belonging to divergent subgroups, suggesting that the two instruments were differently attuned to the various aspects of the presentation of postnatal depression.

Another Welsh study (Thompson et al, 1998) found that the EPDS was superior to the HAD scale in identifying RDC-defined depression and similar to the observer-rated Hamilton Rating Scale for Depression (HRSD; Hamilton, 1960), which it also matched for sensitivity to change in mood over time.

An Australian group (Condon & Corkindale, 1997) found little agreement between the EPDS, the depression sub-scale of the HAD scale, the Zung Self-Rating Depression Scale (SDS; Zung, 1965) and the depression sub-scale of the Profile of Mood States (POMS; McNair & Lorr, 1964). They concluded that this poor level of agreement might reflect the different emphasis in the item content of the questionnaires.

In France, Guedeney et al (2000) compared the EPDS with the GHQ–28 and the Centre for Epidemiological Studies Depression Scale (CES–D; Radloff, 1977), and suggested that the EPDS was better at identifying depression in postnatal women with anhedonic and anxious symptomatology, but less satisfactory for women with psychomotor retardation.

Using a sample of 50 Austrian postnatal women taking part in an international epidemiological study who scored 7 or more on the German version of the EPDS, Muzik et al (2000) compared the EPDS, the German version of the Zung SDS (with a clinical cut-off score of 50), and the depression and anxiety sub-scales of the Symptom Checklist–90–Revised (SCL–90–R; Derogatis & Cleary, 1977) with a cut-off T-score of 63). Diagnoses of depression and anxiety were made using the Structured Clinical Interview for DSM–III–R. The authors reported that the newly developed German version of the EPDS screened reliably for postnatal depression, and that further research was needed to create screening measures for post-partum anxiety disorders.

In the USA, Cheryl Beck (Beck & Gable, 2001) developed a new screening measure, the Post-partum Depression Screening Scale (PDSS). This new scale, developed from qualitative research, was compared with the EPDS and the BDI and validated against a DSM–IV diagnostic interview. She found that the PDSS yielded the highest combination of sensitivity (91%) and specificity (72%) of the three instruments and concluded that researchers and clinicians need to be aware of the differential sensitivity of depression instruments that are supposed to be measuring the same construct. It is also possible that the differences in performance may reflect differences in the population investigated.

We developed the EPDS because other depression measures available at that time were problematic for use with postnatal women living in the community. Other scales may be developed in the future, perhaps specific to a local population, particularly if it is from a diverse cultural background. However, we recommend the continued use of the EPDS because it is so widely used in different countries and therefore allows useful comparison between findings.

Other uses of the EPDS

The EPDS is not specific only to detecting depression in the puerperium. It can also be used to screen for depression in the following: pregnancy (Murray & Cox, 1990; Green & Murray, 1994; Evans et al, 2001; Josefsson et al, 2001); terminal illness (Lloyd-Williams et al, 2000); and fathers (Ballard et al, 1994; Areias et al, 1996b; Matthey et al, 2001). It has been used to assess dysphoria in adoptive parents (Gair, 1999). Cox et al (1996) validated the scale for use with non-postnatal women and it has also been validated for use with the mothers and fathers of toddlers (Thorpe, 1993). The scale can be administered by computer with adequate acceptability and performance (Glaze & Cox, 1991). The EPDS is not a measure of general psychiatric morbidity and will not detect other common perinatal disorders.

CHAPTER 3

International and cultural issues

When establishing a perinatal mental health service it is necessary to take into account the local sociocultural context of childbirth and to recognise that health professionals are required to be culturally competent. The Edinburgh Postnatal Depression Scale (EPDS; Cox *et al*, 1987) can be used inappropriately in research and clinical settings – especially if it has been translated without an adequate validation study having been carried out.

Translation

To our knowledge, the EPDS has been translated into 23 different languages (see Appendix 2, which contains some of the translated versions), and validation studies of the English and many of the translations have been carried out in different countries. The scale can therefore facilitate international research when used as a screening questionnaire and can assist primary care workers to clarify the presence and severity of depressive disorders. It was developed to detect minor as well as major depression: mild depressive symptoms can rapidly escalate into a disabling major depressive disorder. There are important factors to consider when using a translation. The EPDS is not a checklist of symptoms, and it is therefore inappropriate to make cross-cultural comparisons of symptoms or syndromes.

When planning to use the EPDS in an international study it may be helpful, for example, to compare the relative values of an etic approach (when a culture is studied from the outside perspective of a different culture) with the humanistic emic approach, which is derived from an inside understanding, from the perspective of the culture itself. As suggested by Laungani (2000), different assumptions and techniques are often required to understand depression in other cultures and this is just as true for postnatal depression. As Kumar (1994) cogently remarked:

'the way in which the impact (of childbirth) is felt by the individual parent must, to some extent, be shaped by the ways in which that parent's society and culture organises its response to parenthood, as well as by the structure of the family into which the child is born' (p. 250).

In transcultural studies of postnatal depression in Uganda and Scotland (Cox, 1999) the need to understand local folk causes of depression, the range of traditional treatments and the reason for differences in the choice of presenting complaints was self-evident. The Ugandan women were more likely to have somatic symptoms and less likely to express feelings of personal responsibility for the development and nurture of the baby. The range of post-partum support was also strikingly different for African and Scottish women: the Ugandan mothers were part of a much larger family group and a third were co-wives. Naming ceremonies were common in Uganda and was a most important family occasion. They were increasingly rare in Scotland.

When the EPDS is used in another language, especially if that language represents a different worldview, the five areas of equivalence described by Flaherty et al (1988) are of particular importance. These dimensions are:

1.   Content equivalence: the content of each item of the instrument should be relevant to the phenomena of each culture being studied.
2.   Semantic equivalence: the meaning of each item should be the same in each culture after translation into the language and idiom, written or oral, of each culture.
3.   Technical equivalence: the method of assessment (e.g. pencil and paper or interview) should be comparable in each culture with respect to the data that it yields.
4.   Criterion equivalence: the interpretation of the measurement of the variable should remain the same when compared with the norm for each culture studied.
5.   Conceptual equivalence: the instrument should measure the same theoretical construct in each culture.

In a study of depression in Sikh women living in Wolverhampton, in the UK (Clifford et al, 1999), we considered each of these dimensions. To determine semantic equivalence, each EPDS statement (and each word used) was examined to establish whether the meaning and idiom were the same in Punjabi as in English. For technical equivalence, the Punjabi EPDS was tape-recorded to ensure that women who needed verbal rather than written assessment would be approached in the same way.

Validation

The EPDS has been found to have satisfactory validity when translated into most other European languages, although not all such validation studies and translations fully satisfy the five criteria listed above.

Experience to date in an international transcultural project (Oates *et al*, 2003) suggests that in Europe and North and South America the EPDS is useful as a first-stage screening questionnaire, and that it can be administered as described in this handbook.

A list of languages into which the EPDS has been translated, and key references, is given below and some of these translations are included in Appendix 2. Not all of these translations have been validated.

- Arabic (Ghubash *et al*, 1997)
- Chinese (Hong Kong: Lee *et al*, 1998; Taiwan: Heh, 2001)
- Czech (Dragonas *et al*, 1996)
- Dutch (Pop *et al*, 1992)
- French (Guedeney & Fermanian, 1998)
- German (Bergant *et al*, 1998; Muzik *et al*, 2000)
- Greek (Thorpe *et al*, 1992)
- Hebrew (Fisch *et al*, 1997; Glasser & Barell, 1999)
- Hindi (source not known)
- Icelandic (Thome, 1992, 1996, 1999)
- Italian (Carpiniello *et al*, 1997; Benvenuti *et al*, 1999)
- Japanese (Okano *et al*, 1996, 1998)
- Khmer (Fitzgerald *et al*, 1998)
- Konkani (Patel *et al*, 2003)
- Maltese (Felice, 1998)
- Norwegian (Eberhard-Gran *et al*, 2001)
- Portuguese (Areias *et al*, 1996a; Da-Silva *et al*, 1998)
- Punjabi (Clifford *et al*, 1997, 1999)
- Slovenian (M. Blinc Pesek, personal communication, 2003)
- Spanish (Jadresic *et al*, 1995; Vega-Dienstmaier *et al*, 2002)
- Swedish (Lundh & Gyllang, 1993; Wickberg & Hwang, 1996*b*)
- Urdu (source not known)
- Vietnamese (Matthey *et al*, 1997)

No validation study is perfect. A good validation, however, should have an adequate sample size, be representative of the general population, state the time interval between the administration of the EPDS and the clinical interview and indicate that the EPDS has been completed on the basis of the mother's reported feelings in the 7 days preceding its completion. It should also provide details of the method of translation and the background of the researchers and give particular attention to difficulties in translating idioms. Validation studies should also use a culturally appropriate diagnostic interview.

The EPDS deliberately does not contain any somatic items, and this might raise practical problems for local clinicians and research groups if the dominant way in which depression presents is as a physical/ somatic symptom. Social descriptors such as marital status, social class and parenting roles may not be similar in different cultures even within

Europe. In Sweden, for example, the concept of a 'single mother' does not imply that the father is unknown and/or is not providing instrumental and financial support. In Britain, however, being a single mother usually implies that a woman is the sole supporter of her child. In Sweden, it is customary to have a baby baptised. This does not necessarily indicate that a family is religious: it is more a reflection of the fact that until recently Swedish citizens were all registered as members of the State Lutheran Church.

Owing to these and other similar considerations, it is not surprising that validation studies using French (Guedeney & Fermanian, 1998), Chinese (Lee et al, 1998), Swedish (Lundh & Gyllang, 1993; Wickberg & Hwang, 1996), Maltese (Felice, 1998), Italian (Carpiniello et al, 1997; Benvenuti et al, 1999) and Japanese (Okano et al, 1998) translations recommend a lower cut-off score for optimum sensitivity than that found in our original study. These differences may be explained by differing sample sizes or the timing of the post-partum interview and also by difficulties in translating English idioms. For example, in the UK the item 'Things have been getting on top of me' is commonly construed as 'I have felt overwhelmed by everyday tasks or events'. This has a different meaning even in North American English. Again, 'The thought of harming myself has occurred to me' is generally recognised by British women as implying suicidal thoughts, but it could be interpreted as fear of harm occurring through an accident such as falling over.

For such reasons, the use of the EPDS and its technical and conceptual equivalence in Japan, Uganda and in the Punjabi language is not established. There are particular difficulties expressing in Punjabi items referring to anhedonia (the lack of pleasurable anticipation) and the concept of blaming oneself unnecessarily. Importantly, using the EPDS in a culture in which there is uncertainty about the nature of clinical depression and the extent to which it can be reliably assessed may be inappropriate, and could lead to premature recommendations about its effectiveness. Translations of the EPDS need to be tested in new studies to determine their usefulness in research and as a basis for providing services to women in different countries and cultures.

The scale has been used with various populations, such as low-income Brazilian women in Niteroi (Da-Silva et al, 1998) and women following miscarriage in Hong Kong (Lee et al, 1998), and as an outcome measure in a trial of the preventive effectiveness of antenatal information in Japan (Okano et al, 1998). The validated Portuguese translation of the EPDS was used in Porto to investigate the comparative incidence of depression in both fathers and mothers during the woman's pregnancy and after childbirth (Areias et al, 1996a). It is interesting to note that multilingual health workers orally translated the EPDS to women speaking six different South African languages at a postnatal clinic in Johannesburg, where it was validated against DSM–IV (American Psychiatric Association, 1994) criteria for depression (Lawrie *et al*, 1998). In Germany, Bergant *et al* (1998) translated the scale and validated it against ICD–10 (World Health Organization, 1992) criteria for depression at 5 days post-partum in an Innsbruck hospital. Although we consider 5 days to be too soon to administer the scale, the authors reported it to be valid, reliable and 'application friendly' in this language.

The original English version of the scale has been validated for use in North America (O'Hara, 1994: pp. 161–162; Stuart *et al*, 1998), and it is extensively used in Australia, in both research and clinical practice. It has been validated on an Australian sample by Boyce *et al* (1993). Barclay & Kent (1998) have questioned both the use of the EPDS with new immigrant mothers in Australia and the problems of conceptualising extreme misery in this population as 'depression'. They argue that a narrow approach to 'medical aetiology' may fail to include the socio-cultural aspects of postnatal depression experienced by non-English-speaking immigrant women. However, Barnett *et al* (1999), discussing their studies of immigrant Vietnamese and Arabic women in New South Wales, Australia, cogently observed:

'screening for postnatal depression results in more non-English-speaking women being identified and thus offered a service than if such screening does not occur. We disagree with the view that the term "postnatal depression" necessarily implies any aetiology ... Work by our unit, as well as others around the world, indicates that the psychosocial and cultural aspects related to distress in new immigrant mothers is being recognised and acted upon' (p. 203).

CHAPTER 4

Using the Edinburgh Postnatal Depression Scale in clinical settings: research evidence

The following pages include justification for introducing the Edinburgh Postnatal Depression Scale (EPDS; Cox *et al*, 1987) in primary care settings, based on studies that either directly involved health professionals or that have added to our knowledge of the potential use of the EPDS in clinical settings. Further information was derived from training groups of health professionals from different disciplines (including psychologists, psychiatrists and other doctors, community psychiatric nurses, midwives and health visitors) for the introduction of postnatal depression initiatives in the community over the past two decades. Discussions during the training and post-training feedback have provided many valuable insights and added considerably to our knowledge of the practical issues of administering the EPDS.

Routine postnatal screening

It has been suggested that administering the EPDS as a standardised screen with all women is both unnecessary and intrusive. The argument is that experienced health professionals who are in frequent contact with their clients should be able to detect depression without such an aid (see, e.g., Comport, 1990; Barclay & Kent, 1998; Barker, 1998). Both assumptions (acceptability and detection) are challenged by research.

Detection of depression

Let us first consider research evidence concerning detection rates. Health visitors in our counselling intervention (Holden *et al*, 1989) were asked to indicate whether they believed that women in their case-load were experiencing depression at an interview 6 weeks post-partum. The women then completed the EPDS, which they put in a sealed envelope unseen by the health visitors. This study was conducted several years ago in areas where health visitor–client ratios allowed close contact, with weekly visits by the health visitor to mothers with infants under 6 weeks old. Despite knowing the women well, however, the health visitors failed to identify 60% of the 60 women who obtained high EPDS scores at 6 weeks and were subsequently found to have depression at a psychiatric interview at about 3 months post-partum. Other UK researchers (e.g. Angeli & Grahame, 1990; Painter, 1995) reported similar findings. Hearn et al (1998), who set out specifically to determine the efficiency of the primary care team in identifying postnatal depression in women, found that using the EPDS gave an almost three-fold increase in the numbers of women identified with depression.

Many overseas studies have shown that EPDS screening can increase detection rates. In Sweden, where child health care nurses pay regular home visits and where staff:client ratios are considerably better than in the UK, Wickberg & Hwang (1996a) found that health profession-als identified less than half the women found to be depressed in their trial, and that only one-third of the mothers they did identify had spontaneously indicated their feelings. Also working in Sweden, Bågedahl-Strindlund & Monsen Borjesson (1998) found that very few women with postnatal depression are identified in routine care in Sweden. In both Swedish studies, the EPDS was well-accepted by both mothers and nurses, and its use significantly increased the number of identified cases.

Three interesting studies in North America examined the ability of health professionals to detect depression with or without the EPDS. The first is that of Schaper et al (1994), who interviewed physicians and midwives taking part in a community study in Wisconsin. The study aimed to determine the extent of postnatal depression in the selected population and to identify relationships between maternal character-istics and elevated EPDS scores. The authors also wondered whether using the EPDS would increase practitioner awareness and treatment of postnatal depression. Eighty-three per cent of the professionals interviewed reported that the EPDS had increased their awareness of the condition, and 92% had referred patients with high EPDS scores for treatment.

In the second study, based at the Mayo Clinic in Minnesota, Georgiopoulos et al (2001) implemented universal screening with the EPDS in all community postnatal care sites over a 1-year period. The rate of diagnosis of post-partum depression in this community increased from 3.7% before the routine use of EPDS screening to 10.7% following screening. When the medical records of 342 women who had completed an EPDS were reviewed 1 year later, 88 (26%) had been diagnosed as depressed by their general practitioner. All the women who were found to be depressed had received treatment.

In the third study, carried out in Asheville, NC, Evins et al (2000) compared the efficacy of routine clinical evaluation with that of EPDS screening in a residency training programme practice. Over 1 year, 391 patients were assigned either to screening with the EPDS ($n = 79$) or to a control group that had only spontaneous detection during routine clinical evaluation ($n = 96$). These authors reported impressive results:

the incidence of detection of post-partum depression with the EPDS was 35.4%, compared with an incidence of only 6.3% for spontaneous detection during routine clinical evaluation. They concluded that the EPDS is an effective adjunct to clinical interview for diagnosis of post-partum depression and its use should be considered in residency training.

In Sydney, Australia, Barnett et al (1993) asked 100 mothers of infants consecutively admitted to a mothercraft residential facility to complete the EPDS. Of the 100 women who completed an EPDS, 39 (39%) scored above the cut-off point for likely major depressive disorder, only one of whom had been identified prior to the infant's admission as having postnatal depression. Although this study took place several years ago, the authors' words are still relevant:

'The extent of serious mood disorders in the post-partum population has remained generally unacknowledged, despite an upsurge of recent research activity in the field. Nevertheless, this problem has considerable public health significance, impinging as it does on the health of all members of the family' (p. 270).

Acceptability of the EPDS

Do women find the EPDS intrusive or an invasion of their privacy? Although we have heard of isolated instances of individual women being reluctant or even refusing to complete the scale, this has usually been for personal reasons, or because it has been insensitively presented. For example, one woman in our three-centre study felt oppressed by being asked to fill in an EPDS at the baby clinic because she had already been given one at her postnatal visit to the hospital (Gerrard et al, 1994). Another woman was already receiving hospital treatment for depression.

Overall, however, the EPDS has proved its acceptability to women in published studies conducted in a range of different geographical and sociological areas. In the UK, Taylor (1989) in Aberdeen, Cullinan, (1991) in Hertfordshire and Angeli & Grahame (1990) in Walton-on-Thames all reported that most women had no objection to completing the scale. In Cambridge, UK, the EPDS was mailed to 702 women 6 weeks after they had given birth, and the authors concluded that a return rate of 97.3% indicated impressive evidence of the scale's acceptability to the women (Murray & Carothers, 1990).

Researchers in other countries have also reported favourably on both detection rates and the acceptability of the EPDS in clinical studies (e.g. New Zealand: Webster et al (1994) and Holt (1995); Sweden: Lundh & Gyllang (1993) and Wickberg & Hwang (1997); Montreal, Canada: Zelkowitz & Milet (1995); Iceland: Thome (1991)).

In our counselling intervention, when we asked women to comment specifically about their response to the EPDS, the majority reported that it had been a relief to be asked about their feelings. Being asked to complete the questionnaire was usually taken to indicate that the health professional was concerned about their personal well-being and not only about their status as the mother of an infant (Holden, 1991).

Legitimising feelings

Some professionals believe that informing a woman that she is depressed may increase the severity of depressive symptoms, or that she might view the phrase 'postnatal depression' as stigmatising. Elliott (1994) argues cogently:

'Properly explained, 'postnatal depression' labelling, when women are at the bottom of the spiral, may remove 'depression about depression' ... Labelling when at the early depressed mood or subclinical depression level of the spiral may actually create 'depression about depression' if the label is perceived as failure' (p. 223).

Thome (1991) found that Icelandic mothers who scored high on the EPDS did not see their distress as 'mental disturbance', and neither did the nurses who administered the scale and supported them. The nurses in fact admired some for their strength in living through very difficult life situations and not showing more distress than they actually did.

Two studies in primary care showed that depression that has been recognised has a better outcome than that which is missed. Freeling (1992) found that unrecognised depressions last longer, and Ormel *et al* (1990) showed that this is not due to any particular treatment. In a review of therapeutic interventions, Malan *et al* (1975) found that many clients with depression are helped by a single assessment interview. Such improvement may be due to the fact that the person's distress has been shared with and validated by another person (Goldberg, 1992).

'Being told I was depressed helped in so many ways. It meant I could tell other people when they asked how I was. I was amazed how many people said they had had it themselves. Before, I couldn't tell anyone, I just pretended I was fine. I thought no one would understand. But everyone seemed to have a story about someone they had known who was depressed. If everyone was more open about it, people could help each other more' (Holden, 1988: p. 95).

Antenatal research and the EPDS

Many researchers have found that depression is common in pregnancy (e.g. Pitt, 1968; Atkinson & Rickel, 1984; Watson *et al*, 1984; Ancill *et al*, 1986; Gotlib *et al*, 1989; O'Hara *et al*, 1990; Johnstone *et al*, 2001;

Matthey et al, 2001). Green (1998), who presented EPDS scores from 1272 women, found antenatal dysphoria to be at least as prevalent as postnatal and the majority of women had higher EPDS antenatal than postnatal scores. She also maintained that antenatal EPDS scores were fairly good predictors of postnatal scores, as did Josefsson et al (2001).

Many professionals ask whether routine screening would be a useful predictor of postnatal depression, allowing scarce resources to be allocated to those at higher risk. Murray and Cox validated the EPDS for antenatal use in 1990, and it has since been used in several antenatal studies (e.g. Appleby et al, 1994; Green & Murray, 1994) and in the Avon Longitudinal Study of Parents and Children (Evans et al, 2001).

Analysis of the predictive value of an antenatal EPDS is, however, controversial. In contrast to the findings of Green & Murray (1994) and of Josefsson et al (2001) cited above, Evans et al (2001) found that only a small proportion of women are depressed both before and after the birth. In Chile, Jadresic et al (1992) also found that women mainly suffered either antenatal or postnatal depression, but not both. In the UK, Watson et al (1984) and Brugha et al (1998) reported similar findings. A further complication when comparing antenatal and post-natal EPDS scores is that differences that are statistically significant are not necessarily of clinical significance. Matthey (2003) has cogently discussed this important matter and concluded from a review of EPDS validation studies that the Reliable Change Index (RCI) for the EPDS is four points.

So it would seem that there is a large group of women whose postnatal dysphoria is not predictable from antenatal EPDS scores, arguing against the routine use of an antenatal EPDS as a predictor of postnatal depression.

Should the EPDS be used as a routine screen in pregnancy?

It is clear from the research that many pregnant women become depressed; indeed, the Avon study (Evans et al, 2001) found more women to be depressed during pregnancy than after the birth. Detecting depression and offering treatment may be important for both the pregnant mother and her infant and for their future well-being. Recent research suggests that psychopathology may have important effects on the intrauterine environment because of increased cortisol levels (Tcixeira et al, 1999). It may also affect subsequent mothering behaviour: Green & Murray (1994) found that women who had scored high on the EPDS in pregnancy were less likely postnatally either to attempt or to persist with breastfeeding, more likely to view their babies as being 'more difficult' than other babies and more likely to perceive life as more difficult since the birth.

Simply administering the EPDS in pregnancy may have positive benefits. Clark (2000) found that by focusing on the needs of the mother, not only was low emotional well-being identified, but it also provided both clients and health visitors with an opportunity to discuss emotional health, regardless of the antenatal EPDS score.

Other antenatal prediction measures

Measures specifically designed to detect vulnerability factors may also prove effective in predicting depression. Several researchers have developed specific predictive measures, with differing claims of success. Elliott et al (1988) developed one of the earliest of these in a study of the prevention of postnatal depression, although the scale itself has not, to our knowledge, been published.

In Manchester, UK, Appleby and colleagues (Appleby et al, 1994; Warner et al, 1997) developed a 10-item questionnaire based on psycho-social risk factors at 36 weeks. However, although antenatal scores on this questionnaire correlated significantly with EPDS scores at 8 weeks after the birth, the questionnaire failed to discriminate between women who later did or did not become depressed according to psychiatric criteria. The team had more success using a 14-item Maternal Attitudes Questionnaire, based on cognitions relating to role change, expectations of motherhood and expectations of the self as a mother. Maternal Attitudes Questionnaire scores correlated highly with scores on both the EPDS and the Clinical Interview Schedule (Warner et al, 1997).

In Reading, UK, Cooper et al (1996) tested a predictive index on a large sample of 5000 women who had completed an EPDS in the last trimester of pregnancy, and compared the results with the mental state of the women at 6–8 weeks post-partum. The authors claim that their index offers a system for the prediction of post-partum depression that could be of use in both research and clinical practice.

In a Danish study, Nielsen Forman et al (2000) gave an antenatal questionnaire on past history of psychiatric disease, psychological distress and social support to 528 women during pregnancy and compared the results with EPDS scores at 4 months after delivery. They claim that one in three women who suffer from psychological distress in late pregnancy, with perceived social isolation, will develop post-partum depression. Similarly, Webster et al (2000) claimed improved recognition of women at risk of postnatal depression by using an 'objective, psychosocial assessment' (the Maternity Social Support Scale) to screen 901 women antenatally in a hospital-based study in Queensland, Australia.

The overall picture emerging from antenatal screening for postnatal depression suggests that it is helpful to ask women about their emotional state during pregnancy. And, as Green & Murray (1994) point out, organisationally the antenatal care setting in the UK provides ideal opportunities for mass screening: most women attend a hospital clinic at least twice, see their midwife regularly and make several visits to their family doctor.

However, the wide-scale implications must be carefully considered before deciding on routine screening. As with postnatal depression, organisational problems arise after screening, as highlighted in the recommendations of the National Screening Committee in the UK (see Adams, 2002). Who decides whether the woman should be further assessed and by whom? What treatment should she receive and who will administer this and supervise her care? For pregnant women with severe depression, do the benefits of antidepressants outweigh the risks? It is important that further research is carried out to study the potential benefits and problems.

Identifying pregnant women at risk of developing puerperal psychosis

A most important task for midwives is not just to screen for current antenatal depression, but also to identify women at high risk of developing a puerperal psychosis. These are women with a past history of psychosis, for whom there is a 1 in 4 risk of developing a further psychosis. Also at risk are women with a family or personal history of severe depression, in particular 'manic' or bipolar depression.

It was pointed out by Margaret Oates in *The Confidential Enquiries into Maternal Deaths in the United Kingdom* (Oates, 2001) that women with a history of severe mental disorders are often incorrectly categorised as having previous postnatal depression. This may lead to underestimation of the likely severity of a recurrence.

It is for this reason that simply administering the EPDS routinely at the booking-in clinical is not recommended. Rather, specific and sensitive inquiry should be made about previous psychiatric history. In particular, if the woman says that she had postnatal depression following a previous birth, the severity of the episode must be ascertained. As Oates (2001) points out:

'most women who have experienced a previous severe post-partum mental illness will be concerned about future recurrence. All those involved, midwives, obstetricians, GPs and psychiatrists need to acquire knowledge of the high risk of recurrence, and to know that women with early onset conditions can quickly move from appearing to be merely anxious and depressed to being psychotic and suicidal within a few days. They also need to know that being mentally well during pregnancy does not necessarily reduce the risk of recurrence following delivery.

Psychiatric, midwifery and obstetric staff need to communicate with each other and with the general practitioner verbally and in writing about the care of women during pregnancy who are at risk of a post-partum mental illness' (p.186).

Conclusions from EPDS screening research

The EPDS is clearly being used in many ways and in many different contexts throughout the world. Research suggests that its use by health professionals can help them to identify both postnatal and antenatal depression. However, a large-scale study of the effectiveness of EPDS screening has not yet been carried out. These issues are further discussed in Chapter 6, in which the problems of introducing a postnatal depression service are outlined.

There are those who rightly criticise an over-systematised regime. In an article entitled 'Let's trust our instincts', Barker (1998) pointed out that health professionals should be encouraged to use their experience, insight and intuition, rather than simply relying on predetermined formulae to assess the well-being of their clients. However, as Taylor (1998) observed, 'relying on Walter Barker's somewhat sentimental ideas of intuition merely assists the de-skilling process that he says he is trying to prevent' (p. 427).

Most clinical studies have concluded that the majority of women readily accept routine use of the EPDS. However, it is important to realise that all were confidential research projects or sensitive innovative clinical studies. To date there have been no published studies of women's responses in non-research settings. Women's willingness to disclose personal information will, of course, be influenced by their perception of how that information will be used and who will have access to it.

Clinical psychologists Angela Leviston and Maria Downs argue that instinct is not enough, maintaining that if used properly the scale can enhance clinical practice (Leviston & Downs, 1999). This point cannot be overemphasised. As Elliott & Leverton (2000) cogently point out in a review article:

'The EPDS is clearly not a magic wand to be distributed for compulsory use without training. Alone it is just a piece of paper, a checklist. Combined with training in prevention, detection and treatment, however, it becomes an important part of an effective programme' (p. 303).

CHAPTER 5

Counselling and other psychotherapeutic intervention in perinatal depression

Various studies over the past two decades have looked at ways of treating or preventing postnatal depression. Clinical research is by no means easy, particularly when it involves health professionals in changes to their normal practice, and no intervention trials are perfect. Results are, however, encouraging, and innovative research has produced many ideas that could be adapted for use in clinical practice.

The Edinburgh counselling intervention

The Edinburgh counselling intervention (Holden *et al*, 1989) gave health visitors a key role in helping to find practical ways of helping women with depression in a randomised controlled trial of counselling. The process leading to the implementation of this study is described here in detail for the first time, because we believe that it has implications both for research and for the introduction of perinatal depression programmes into health service provision. In particular, it highlights the importance of preliminary liaison and discussion between primary care and mental health services.

Outline of the study

Seventeen health visitors in Edinburgh and Livingston (Scotland) were given brief training in the principles of non-directive counselling and in how to administer the Edinburgh Postnatal Depression Scale (EPDS; Cox *et al*, 1987). Women who had scored 12 or above 6 weeks after giving birth were assessed for depression during a home visit about 3 months after the birth by a research psychiatrist using the Clinical Interview Schedule (Goldberg *et al*, 1970), with the diagnosis of depression derived from the Research Diagnostic Criteria (Spitzer *et al*, 1978). Women with depression were randomly allocated to the treatment group or to a control group who received routine primary care. Health visitors were only informed of women in the treatment group, who received eight weekly visits in their own home, when they were encouraged to talk about their feelings; questions about baby care were discussed separately. The health visitors were asked to counsel only those women referred to them and to complete a research form for each session. The research psychiatrist, who was given no information regarding the group to which each woman had been allocated, reassessed the women at home after 3 months. Our main finding was that 18 of the 27 counselled women showed no depression at the second interview, whereas only 9 of the 23 women who had received routine treatment had recovered. The percentages of recovered women in the counselled and control groups were 69.2% and 37.7% respectively. The difference, 31.7%, had a 95% confidence interval of 5–58%. The chi-squared statistic was 5.06, with one degree of freedom and an associated P of 0.03.

What we discovered   positive effect visit

We learned from this study that giving health visitors information about postnatal depression and instructions in using the EPDS and non-directive counselling could have a positive impact on the lives of women with postnatal depression. Confiding their feelings to their health visitor during counselling significantly reduced depressive symptoms. There were also other benefits: in tape-recorded interviews 10–12 months postnatally, many counselled women reported beneficial effects on their relationship with their partner and changes in their perception of the health visitor's role. Counselled women were more likely to view the health visitor as being there for them as well as for the baby, whereas women in the control group were less likely to see their health visitor as someone in whom they could confide.

Counselled women whose depression remained after counselling ('non-recovered counselled women') nevertheless benefited from the intervention, as demonstrated by their subsequent help-seeking be-haviour. For all the women we found to be depressed at the first and second interviews we informed the family doctors of our findings. Women who were still depressed at the second interview were advised to consult their doctor. The women's medical records were examined and their family doctors were asked about their progress a year later. Seventy-five per cent of the non-recovered counselled women had sought medical help, compared with only 13% of non-recovered controls. The attention of their health visitor may have encouraged counselled women to view their depression as a legitimate reason to consult, and having their depression validated may also have increased compliance with treatment. It was, however, disappointing that the family doctors had not sought contact with women who were still depressed after the study period, but had left it to the women themselves to seek further help.

We gained useful information about the EPDS. During the 2.5 years it took to collect our data, the scale was administered routinely at about

6 weeks postnatally to all women attending baby clinics in the five participating health centres. Although the research team undertook responsibility for scoring the EPDS and deciding on eligibility for entering the trial, the health visitors were nevertheless involved in considerable changes. They reported that most women readily accepted screening and that with some readjustments to clinic procedures, administration could be absorbed into routine practice. An added reported advantage was that use of the scale resulted in a general raising of awareness among all members of the primary health care team, and also among the women themselves and their families, of the possibility of emotional distress or depression occurring at this time and of the importance of providing the opportunity for women to talk about their feelings.

Setting up the study

This positive response of health professionals and mothers to what was at that time a complete departure from their previous practice was most encouraging. It should be pointed out, however, that the changes did not just happen from one day to the next. It took 6 months of preliminary negotiations, meetings and discussion before we agreed on policy and before EPDS screening was introduced. All members of the primary care team were involved in the decision-making, as also were community psychiatrists and community psychiatric nurses, as well as the ethics committee and nursing managers. After the family doctors and nursing management had given their permission for the research to take place, the final decision was left to the health visitors, who were given a month to decide whether or not they wished to participate. For research purposes, it had to be a case of 'one in, all in' in each of the five health centres, and there were many, sometimes heated, debates. Their decision-making was centred on the knowledge we had all gained during the lengthy preliminary discussions and anxieties about the extra work that would be involved for them (EPDS screening and extra visits to women in the counselled group) and about the counselling itself. Finally, all the health centres we had approached agreed to participate.

Training the health visitors

We were allocated three 2-hour time slots by management for the training, and these sessions were held weekly in each of the health centres. In the sessions we covered the practical details of the administration of the EPDS. The questionnaires were to be completed by mothers at the 6-week baby clinic visit, then placed by the mother in a sealed envelope with scores unseen by the health visitor and posted in a box for collection. We also discussed the importance of sensitivity in introducing the EPDS to the women, and the information to be given to the women (who also each received a formal letter inviting their participation in the research). Other important topics included ethical considerations and the philosophy and practical guidelines for the non-directive counselling we had decided upon.

These meetings were dynamic rather than didactic, although information was, of course, provided. Ruth Sagovsky (a research psychiatrist) and Jeni Holden (the project organiser and trainer of the health visitors) had made two simple videos, which provoked lively discussion of the 'dos and don'ts' of counselling and possible conflicts that could arise between the role of health visitor and that of counsellor. We also provided written material to be read between sessions. However, even before this short training commenced, we had covered many important issues in our previous exploratory meetings.

So, before embarking on our research intervention, the health visitors and doctors were as fully informed as it was possible to be in the light of this innovatory experiment. We were all, at this time, pioneers. Jeni Holden visited each of the health centres weekly during the course of the research, to collect the completed EPDS forms and to discuss any problems that the health visitors were experiencing, either with counselling or with the administration of the EPDS. These problems were resolved on an ad hoc basis. These visits provided an informal support for the health visitors and valuable information regarding the feasibility of the system.

Problems

Once the study was under way we experienced surprisingly few problems, considering the changes being made to normal practice. This may have been due to our lengthy preliminary discussions and the involvement of all members of each primary care team. The health visitors had all 'opted in', and were enthusiastic about their part in the research. They did not have responsibility for making decisions about treatment, and at our weekly support meetings they were able to diffuse any anxieties.

Extending research findings into clinical practice

A three-centre trial of health visitor training for postnatal depression was undertaken in London, Edinburgh and Stoke-on-Trent (Gerrard et al, 1994; Elliott et al, 2001). The training was based on findings from our own previous counselling study (Holden et al, 1989) and from a trial of the prevention of postnatal depression by Elliott *et al* (1988). Our aim was to share what had been learned about the prevention, identification and treatment of postnatal depression and to give health visitors the opportunity to decide which aspects to adopt in their own work. Training included use of the EPDS and information about non-directive counselling and prevention, which evolved from our counselling study (Holden *et al*, 1989), with the inclusion of preventive measures derived from the study by Elliott *et al* (1988). The health visitors were encouraged to develop strategies based on local resources and to visit women in late pregnancy, to inform them about the study and about the possibility of depression. Training was carried out during seven 2-hour training sessions delivered fortnightly and then monthly. Most groups also had three further monthly sessions with topics suggested by the health visitors, so they were well supported while setting up the service. Again, preliminary meetings were held with doctors, nursing management and the psychiatric team to decide on clear lines of referral for women whose depressions were severe or resistant to simple measures.

As the timing of onset of depression may differ, the EPDS was to be given on three occasions: at 6–8 weeks, 10–12 weeks and about 6 months after the birth, to fit in with normal contact times. The health visitors were asked to visit women who obtained scores of 12 or above 2 weeks later, when they would be asked to complete another EPDS. Those who again scored above threshold would be advised to see their family doctor and, if appropriate, offered a set number of 'listening visits' from the health visitor before review.

There were more problems in this extended trial of training, perhaps understandably, as the health visitors were being asked to take considerably more responsibility and to do even more extra work than in our previous trial. Although, as before, each health centre was approached and the health visitors were invited to take part, not all 'opted in' unreservedly: some were persuaded by management to participate. The health visitors found administration of the three screenings more time-consuming and had trouble remembering when they were due. These problems were addressed by printing the three forms in different colours: blue for EPDS1, pink for EPDS2, yellow for EPDS3. The forms for each mother came with the child record card, and when each EPDS was completed, the health visitor transferred the score to a separate record sheet, and then sent the forms to the research team. However, as we did not receive complete data for every woman, screening on three different occasions was probably asking too much of the service. The health visitors reported that administration was complicated and that although the majority of women were happy to comply with the first screening, some mothers who were not depressed were reluctant to complete even a second EPDS.

What we learned from the three-centre trial: relevance to clinical practice

Our expectation, derived from our original study (i.e. that the health visitors could themselves take responsibility for treatment decisions based on EPDS scores followed by 8 weeks of counselling), was over-optimistic. As Elliott pointed out:

'The knowledge that a second high EPDS score is a good predictor of psychiatric diagnosis of depression, treatable by counselling, was not sufficient to make health visitors confident about their role in "decision to treat" in individual cases' (Elliott, 1994: p. 229).

In our original study, the research psychiatrist made the decision to treat, and the health visitors were asked only to give the 'counselling package' to women we referred to them, that is, to only half of the women in their case-load whom we had found to be depressed. Thus, not only did they have less responsibility, they also had fewer women to counsel.

Also, some health visitors were uncomfortable with the term 'counselling', arguing that our brief training did not qualify them as counsellors. We therefore changed the terminology to 'listening visits'.

It became clear that the referral systems needed to be clarified. In Edinburgh, we already had 3 years of groundwork from the previous study; the psychiatric services were aware of our work and had agreed on a referral system. The health visitors could contact a community psychiatric nurse directly, who would accompany them on a home visit to women about whom they were concerned, with a view to further referral if required. In Stoke-on Trent, they could refer women directly to the Charles Street Parent and Baby Day Unit (Cox *et al*, 1993). In London, however, a specialist psychiatrist needed to be appointed, as there was no pre-existing referral system.

On the basis of our experiences during this study, we concluded that 'for health visitors it may be better to shift from the notion of "selection for treatment" to what is almost prevention' (Elliott, 1994: p. 229) – which is, of course, part of their job description. Offering 2–4 listening visits on the basis of a high score at the first EPDS can, Elliott suggests, prevent the spiral into diagnosable depression. Women whose scores remain high should be referred to psychiatric services.

In the three-centre trial (Gerrard *et al*, 1994; Elliott *et al*, 2001), health visitors were trained in prevention of postnatal depression, EPDS administration, counselling intervention and psychiatric liaison. Before training commenced, the health visitors were asked to give an EPDS to all women in their case-loads at 6 months postnatal as a baseline. During the training trial, other women completed an EPDS at regular intervals.

A comparison of women's EPDS scores at 6 months postnatally before and after training in Stoke-on-Trent showed that participation in the programme enabled health visitors to influence positively the postnatal emotional well-being of women in their case-load, evidenced by a highly significant reduction in mean EPDS scores and in the numbers of women who scored above threshold (Gerrard *et al*, 1994; Elliott *et al*, 2001). On recent enquiry, Edinburgh health visitors were still using EPDS screening and offering listening visits to women with postnatal depression.

The Cambridge intervention trials

Because of a mounting body of evidence of the adverse effects of maternal depression on infants' cognitive and emotional development, Murray and her colleagues embarked on a trial comparing three different psychosocial interventions administered by either a health visitor or a trained psychotherapist. As in our own counselling intervention (Holden *et al*, 1989), the health visitors and therapists had no responsibility for assessment or treatment decisions. Women in the Cambridge study were assessed for depression using a preliminary postal EPDS (scored by researchers) followed by a standardised psychiatric interview.

The four randomly assigned conditions were: non-directive counselling; cognitive–behavioural therapy directed at problems of infant management such as feeding and sleeping; brief dynamic psychotherapy centred on the mother–infant relationship; and routine primary care. The EPDS and psychiatric interview were used to measure recovery from depression; effects on mother–infant interactions were assessed by videotaped interactions. Cooper & Murray (1997) reported a significant effect from all three brief interventions on speed of recovery from depression and on the quality of infants' attachment to recovered mothers. Early remission from depression, itself significantly related to receiving treatment, was associated with a reduced rate of insecure attachments. Importantly, there were no differences in outcome between either the type of intervention or whether therapy was delivered by a trained psychotherapist or a health visitor.

This study led to a further intervention trial in which all Cambridge health visitors were taught to use a combination of counselling and cognitive–behavioural interventions at home-based visits, using the EPDS (administered by the health visitors) to assess depression and monitor recovery. Levels of dysphoria and mothers' reports of relationship problems with their infants improved significantly compared with the control group who received only routine treatment. After training, health visitors effected substantial improvements compared with the pre-training period. The authors claimed that results from both of these studies show that health visitors who have been trained in the use of the EPDS and in the management and detection of postnatal depression can provide help that is both effective and acceptable to mothers (Seeley *et al*, 1996; Cooper & Murray, 1997; Murray *et al*, 2003).

Health visitor counselling in Sweden

Wickberg & Hwang (1996*a*) also conducted a randomised trial of non-directive counselling based on our own study. They identified a sample of 57 women with depression, using EPDS screening at 8 and 12 weeks and the Montgomery–Åsberg Depression Rating Scale (MADRS) and DSM–III–R at about 13 weeks post-partum. Of these, 41 agreed to participate and were randomly allocated to counselling or a control group. Those in the study group received 6 weekly counselling visits by the child health clinic nurse and the control group received routine primary care. Twelve (80%) of the 15 women with major depression in the study group were fully recovered after the intervention, compared with 4 (25%) of the 16 with major depression in the control group.

In a personal communication (2001) Birgitta Wickberg informed us that the Swedish National Council for Medical Research has recommended the implementation of postnatal screening and intervention throughout Sweden. Almost all child health care centres have a consultant psychologist, who will train and offer regular supervision to the staff.

Comparing antidepressant therapy and cognitive counselling

Appleby *et al* (1997) conducted a controlled trial with the antidepressant drug fluoxetine and cognitive–behavioural counselling in Manchester, UK. In a randomised sample of 61 women found to be depressed at 6–8 weeks postnatally, the group compared fluoxetine with placebo treatment, with counselling (both a single session and six sessions) and with combinations of drugs and counselling. The cognitive counselling was designed to be delivered by non-specialists in mental health (e.g. health visitors), after a brief training. All subjects received one session of counselling, and the team were able to compare the additional benefits of the antidepressant and/or additional counselling sessions. A psychiatrist blind to the treatment group measured assessment of recovery on the basis of mean scores and 95% confidence limits on the Clinical Interview Schedule – Revised, the EPDS and the Hamilton Rating Scale for Depression.

Highly significant improvement was seen in all four treatment groups, the fluoxetine group showing significantly greater improvement than those receiving placebo. Improvement after six sessions of counselling was significantly greater than after a single session, but the interaction between counselling and fluoxetine was not statistically significant. The authors concluded that both fluoxetine and cognitive–behavioural counselling are effective treatments for non-psychotic postnatal depression in women and that the women might therefore themselves make the choice of treatment.

These results are promising, although generalisability is tempered by the fact that the numbers in each treatment cell were small. Of the 188 women with depression who were invited to participate, 101 refused, mainly because of the possibility of being allocated to the drug therapy group, and a further 9 dropped out during the trial because of adverse side-effects. Also, although the cognitive–behavioural counselling was designed to be administered by health visitors with a brief training in the method, it has not yet been demonstrated whether this would be practicable and effective in routine health care practice.

In our experience, many women with severe depression post-partum require a combination of treatment with antidepressant medication and appropriate psychotherapy. However, as the Appleby et al (1997) study shows, many women are reluctant to take drug therapy postnatally. It could be an important task for a health professional to explain the effects and benefits of antidepressants and to encourage compliance with medication. For a full discussion of the use of antidepressants and other psychotrophic drugs for breast-feeding women, see Wisner et al (1996) and Stein (1998). More studies are urgently required of the effectiveness of antidepressant therapy in this context.

Interpersonal psychotherapy

O'Hara et al (2000) describe a randomised controlled trial of inter-personal psychotherapy with women in North America meeting DSM–IV criteria for postnatal depression. Sixty per cent of those who received 12 sessions of interpersonal psychotherapy showed a significant improvement, compared with only 20% of waiting-list controls. Therapy was conducted by 10 trained psychotherapists, who each read specified manuals and received 40 hours of didactic lectures and training. Although this is an innovative study, such an intervention would not normally be available to many in the British National Health Service.

Telephone counselling

Thome & Alder (1999) claim successful results from a randomised controlled trial of a telephone intervention in Iceland to reduce fatigue and its resulting distress symptoms in 78 Icelandic mothers who reported having a behaviourally difficult infant 2–3 months of age. This simple intervention could be tried in health service provision.

Group interventions in postnatal depression

Clinical psychologist Jeanette Milgrom and her colleagues reported positive outcomes from a trial comparing different psychotherapeutic approaches with depressed postnatal women in a hospital setting in Melbourne, Australia (Milgrom et al, 1999). In their study, which is still underway, six to eight women participate in groups led by two trained psychotherapists using a cognitive–behavioural approach based on work by Lewinsohn et al (1984) and Olioff (1991).

Psychotherapy, cognitive therapy and couple counselling

Bryanne Barnett and her colleagues in Sydney, Australia (Morgan et al, 1997) described a group programme for postnatally distressed women and their partners that consists of eight sessions, including one session for the couple. Psychotherapeutic and cognitive–behavioural strategies were used to help the women deal with concerns such as their anxieties and feelings towards their partners, their own mothers and their infants. The programme also encourages the men to provide emotional and practical support to their partner. Interestingly, although the programme was successful over time in reducing maternal distress and increasing mothers' self-esteem, about half of the men showed elevated levels of distress.

In a small study in British Columbia, Misri et al (2000) conducted a randomised controlled trial of partner support with 29 women who met DSM–IV criteria for postnatal depression. The support group consisted of women and their partners, with only women in the control group. The patients in both groups were each seen for seven psychoeducational visits; partners in the support group took part in four of the seven visits. Depressive symptoms in the support group women decreased significantly, as measured by the General Health Questionnaire and the EPDS. The authors concluded that partner support has a measurable effect on women experiencing postnatal depression.

Massage and support groups

Onozawa et al (2001) in London tried regular infant massage classes to reduce maternal depression and improve the quality of mother–infant interaction. Thirty-four mothers with first-time depression were randomly allocated either to an infant massage class and support group or to a control support group for five weekly sessions from about 9 weeks postnatally. EPDS scores fell in both groups, but significant improvements in mother–infant interaction (assessed by videotape ratings) were seen only in the massage group. The sample size was small and the authors were unable to distinguish which aspects of the massage class contributed to the benefit, but concluded that learning infant massage is an effective way of facilitating mother–infant interaction.

Health-visitor-led support/therapy groups

Group support or group therapy is likely to be helpful as the woman starts to recover. In the early stages of depression, most women need the nurture provided by a one-to-one relationship and many find it threatening to attend a group. They may also have difficulty organising themselves to get out of the house, which could intensify their feelings of failure if group therapy was the only resource offered. Readers should note that running therapy groups is a specialist and time-consuming area that requires expertise: it should not be attempted without input from trained personnel. Many health visitors have, however, combined with community psychiatric nurses to set up successful groups (e.g. Eastwood, 1995; Pitts, 1995).

Day hospital care

North Staffordshire, in the UK, is uniquely favoured by having a psychiatric day unit for mothers with postnatal depression and their babies (Cox et al, 1993). The atmosphere is informal and welcoming, and the underlying philosophy is that many cases are likely to have psychosocial origins. Members of the multi-disciplinary team are trained in non-directive counselling and are also familiar with the range of antidepressant medication. Cognitive therapy is available from a clinical psychologist. Activities offered include yoga, meditation, individual and group therapy, relaxation, a stress-management group, assertiveness training and creative therapy (including art and role-play).

Boath et al (1999) compared 30 women treated at the North Staffordshire facility with 30 women who received routine primary care. Clinical, marital and social adjustment were measured using the EPDS, the Clinical Interview Schedule, the Anxiety sub-scale of the Hamilton Rating Scale for Depression, the Dyadic Adjustment Scale and the Work Leisure and Family Life Scale. At baseline the groups were similar, but there were significant differences in outcome at 3- and 6-month follow-up for all measures except the Dyadic Adjustment Scale. Doctors and health visitors were informed of any women in the primary care treatment group who were depressed and of the progress of the women in both groups. The team anticipated that:

'providing these professionals with a diagnosis would influence treatment and hence improve clinical outcome ... our findings suggest that being told that a woman has postnatal depression does not in itself lead to effective treatment' (Boath *et al*, 1999: p. 150).

These findings echoed our own disappointment with the lack of doctor-initiated follow-up care provided to women who had taken part in our counselling study. As the authors point out, this indicates a need to train doctors to screen for postnatal depression and to treat it. These issues are further dicussed in Chapter 6.

Antenatal interventions

Little research has yet been done in the treatment of antenatal depression, although Yonkers & Little (2001) provide a helpful overview of the management of psychiatric disorders in pregnancy.

Non-pharmacological interventions that have been shown to be effective in postnatal depression (e.g. listening visits and cognitive therapy), perhaps administered by midwives and health visitors, could usefully be evaluated for their effectiveness in treating depression in pregnancy. In a large prospective study in which the EPDS was administered by midwives, Green & Murray (1994) reported that the women at greatest risk of continuing depression were those with poor marital relationships and no one to talk to. The researchers were encouraged to find that midwives were responding with significantly more home visits to such women. In a recent large controlled study of enhanced midwifery practice which involved over 2000 women, 36 general practice clusters in the West Midlands (UK) were randomly allocated to intervention ($n=17$) or routine treatment ($n=19$). Midwives in both groups attended a study day and those in the intervention group received extra training in the new model of care. Symptom checklists and the EPDS were used to identify individual needs and guidelines were given to the midwives for the management of these needs. Care was extended to 28 days, with a discharge consultation at 10–12 weeks. The redesigned community postnatal care package was associated with improved mental health outcomes for the index group, including reduction in EPDS scores (MacArthur *et al*, 2002).

This study suggests an extended role for midwives in the emotional well-being of women in their care and the importance of including midwives in developing a local perinatal mental health strategy, as recommended by the Royal College of Psychiatrists (2000).

In the few studies of intervention for antenatal depression that have been reported, psychotherapy has been the treatment of choice. Spinelli (1997) piloted a treatment programme with 13 women with major antenatal depression that used interpersonal psychotherapy. She recorded a reduction in depressive symptoms over the 16 weeks of the trial. This study was extended as a controlled clinical treatment trial which is still ongoing. In another interesting naturalistic study, Steinberg and colleagues (Steinberg et al, 1999) conducted a longitudinal prospective study involving pregnant women, 91 of whom had depression and 45 of whom were not depressed; the study continued over 6 months into the postnatal period. They used individual psychotherapy, combining strategies from interpersonal and cognitive–behavioural psychotherapy and/or marital interventions and pharmacology.

Although depressive symptoms (measured by the EPDS and the Hamilton Rating Scale for Depression) in the index group generally improved by the second to third month of treatment, marital discord and child care stress levels did not. The authors concluded that although short-term interventions are a cost-effective way of dealing with depression, 'creative solutions are required to extend treatment sufficiently to address couple conflicts and facilitate the transition to parenthood'.

A few antenatal interventions have been directed towards prevention, with ideas that could be incorporated into existing systems of antenatal classes and/or postnatal support groups. Two simple early studies are still worthy of note. First, over 40 years ago Gordan & Gordan (1960) added two 40-minute sessions to traditional antenatal classes, in which women and their partners were advised to seek information and practical help, to make friends with couples experienced in childcare, to avoid moving house, to get plenty of rest, to discuss plans and worries, to cut down unnecessary activities and to arrange baby-sitters. They reported that women who were encouraged during pregnancy to confide in their husbands and enlist their practical help not only did get more help, but also were less likely to become depressed. Second, in the 1970s Shereshefsky & Lockman (1973) showed that the marital relationships of women who received individual antenatal counselling about the possible effect of childbirth on their relationship remained stable, whereas those in a control group had deteriorated by 6-months post-partum.

Antenatal support and information groups

Elliott et al (1988) invited pregnant women who had been identified as being vulnerable to developing depression to informal locally based antenatal groups designed to give professional support and information about coping strategies during pregnancy and after the birth. The groups also provided the opportunity to meet other women and develop peer-group support. Although attendance among second-time mothers was low, and the numbers in this study were small, at 6 months after delivery the invited first-time mothers showed only half the prevalence of postnatal depression found in non-invited mothers.

Other preventive interventions have, however, proved less successful. In Adelaide, Australia, Stamp *et al* (1995) invited women who had been identified as vulnerable using the Modified Antenatal Screening Questionnaire to support groups that met during pregnancy and continued postnatally. The control group had no intervention. Sadly, attendance at their groups was low, and the intervention did not reduce postnatal depression. They concluded that using groups separate from the standard antenatal classes may have affected attendance, and that more research is required into ways of reaching and supporting women who may become depressed.

Brugha and his colleagues in Leicester, England, conducted a larger trial (Brugha *et al*, 2000). Their programme 'Preparing for parenthood' was designed to increase social support and improve problem-solving skills. Of the 1300 pregnant women originally screened, outcome data were obtained from 190 at 3 months postnatally. Forty-five per cent of the intervention-group women had attended sufficient sessions to be likely to benefit if the intervention was effective. However, this intervention was not effective in preventing depression, and attenders derived no more benefit than non-attenders. The authors concluded that further research is needed.

Other ways of helping during the perinatal period

Many of the studies discussed in this chapter contain ideas and strategies that health professionals may be able to adapt in their own practice. There are, however, other simple ways of helping women during the perinatal period. Primary care workers are, for example, ideally placed to put women in touch with others in a similar situation and to encourage 'befriending' of newcomers or women who have perhaps been at work and do not know many other women in their locality. Information exchange and support groups can be facilitated in antenatal clinic waiting rooms by the provision of a friendly atmosphere and cups of tea.

Liaison with other agencies

Health professionals are usually familiar with other forms of help that may be available locally and encourage women to utilise them. In the UK, for example, one empowering scheme is Homestart, a voluntary home-visiting programme with over 100 branches. Homestart works closely with both statutory and voluntary agencies, and has paid organisers and secretaries, and volunteers who have been 'realistically recruited, carefully prepared, sensitively matched with only one or two families at a time, and meticulously supported' (Harrison, 1992). Volunteers offer friendship, support and practical help to young families experiencing difficulties for up to 2 years after the birth of their child, acting as a friend and confidant, and helping to build self-confidence in using other services. Self-help groups can also increase mothers' self-confidence by giving them the opportunity to discuss shared experiences. MAMA, the Meet-a-Mum Association, offers informal home-based groups for mothers who feel isolated after the birth (see Holden, 1994b).

In Australia, the Post and Ante Natal Depression Association (PaNDa) performs a similar function and the excellent work of the Tresillian Family Centre is well known. Cry-sis is a rather specialised association for parents whose babies cry excessively, with groups and telephone contacts throughout the UK. The Association for Postnatal Illness has had an important role in publicising postnatal depression and in helping individual women by giving them a telephone supporter. Women who have benefited from such help often go on to become volunteer helpers themselves. Alternative therapies such as relaxation, aromatherapy or art therapy may also be available locally. Before setting up a postnatal depression programme, it is useful to inform local voluntary agencies of the proposed project and to enlist their help.

Partners and the extended family

Partners and the extended family are often puzzled as to how best to care for a woman with postnatal depression. They will be able to offer more constructive help if they are informed about the condition and useful strategies. Routine contacts in health centre settings can provide opportunistic teaching and support sessions, and the waiting room is an ideal place for explanatory posters and leaflets. An updated list of information about facilities available in the area is also valuable. Pace (1992) described a health education library in general practice with 400 books in the waiting room for patients to 'dip into' or borrow. Books on mental health and childcare were the most popular.

There is clearly a wide range of ways in which perinatal women and their partners can be helped to enjoy this precious time with a new infant. In a recent review of the postnatal literature, Boath & Henshaw (2001) concluded:

'Based on the variable success of the interventions ... and the premise that postnatal depression results from a multitude of individual and contextual factors, it is feasible that no single intervention can treat all episodes of postnatal depression. Thus a multi-faceted, integrated approach, involving links between the formal and informal services that are currently available, collaboration between primary care professionals and community and secondary psychiatric staff, and patient education and involvement, that would allow women to choose the intervention(s) most relevant to their needs should be explored' (p. 243).

Strategies most likely to succeed are those that lead to empowerment and increased feelings of self-worth for the individual. Many promising studies have already been conducted, and there is evidence of continuing research into innovations in health care. However, long-term follow-up studies will be needed to demonstrate the true effectiveness of early interventions.

CHAPTER 6

Edinburgh Postnatal Depression Scale screening and intervention services

'I wouldn't mind the morning sickness or the actual birth of the baby, it is the postnatal depression that really frightens me. I don't think I could face that again. It was horrific.'

(A mother's comment during interview)

The consequences of maternal depression are costly not only on a personal level, but also in terms of health service resources, including money as well as personnel. It is therefore important that services should be relevant, targeted and research-based. The fact that women's contact with health professionals is at a peak around the time of childbirth provides an ideal opportunity for intervention and for ensuring that these contacts are used with maximum efficiency to meet the needs of individual women.

As discussed in an earlier chapter, research consistently shows that even where contact between professionals and mothers is high, detection of postnatal depression is low. Failure to diagnose depression may be due to short appointments, a physical orientation of care and an emphasis on the baby's rather than the mother's well-being. During the first 6 weeks after the birth, postnatal depression may be hard to differentiate from the normal adjustment to the infant, but by the end of this period health care input normally lessens. In today's economic climate, regular home visits may be increasingly difficult to achieve.

Edinburgh Postnatal Depression Scale (EPDS; Cox *et al*, 1987) screening by primary care staff as part of a well-constructed programme of perinatal care can, we believe, lead to increased detection rates and improved outcomes. The scale can, however, be misused if it is administered without prior explanation by busy professionals who have not been trained in its use and without the full support of health managers and interdisciplinary colleagues. In 1991 a conference was held at Keele in the UK to discuss the increasing use (and misuse) of the EPDS. One session was devoted to a workshop led by Sandra Elliott, comparing models developed in health visiting practice. In her report she wrote:

'The EPDS is a short and simple tool. Its introduction into primary care is anything but simple. In its wake it carries widespread system change as well as a new philosophy' (Elliott, 1994: p. 229).

An audit was carried out in Oxford, UK, to study the effectiveness of services delivered to postnatal women in 26 out of 32 general practices by examining data about routine screening with the EPDS at about 6–8 weeks and at 8 months (Shakespeare, 2002). Health visitors in the area had been trained by a psychiatrist and a psychologist who had completed a 'training for trainers' course (Gerrard *et al*, 1994). Shakespeare found that only 66% of women were screened at 6–8 weeks and this dropped to 55% at 8 months. Although health visitors shared a commitment to this time-consuming and challenging work, there were problems. For example, record-keeping was not standardised; women from ethnic minorities were not being reached; some women refused to complete an EPDS; and different practices achieved different levels of screening. It was considered that workloads in deprived areas may be dispro-portionately high, presentation of the EPDS may differ from one practice to another, and resource and training issues were also identified. This study showed that even with a strategic approach to screening for postnatal depression, only a proportion of women are actually screened and two major issues were raised: first, whether screening for postnatal depression is realistic in practice, especially in deprived areas with a heavy workload; and second, whether the way in which the EPDS is offered affects a woman's willingness to fill it in.

Both of these are important considerations. In areas where health visitors are already overstretched, EPDS screening could be seen as an additional and unwelcome responsibility. However, most of the health visitors J. H. has worked with as colleagues or as trainees have said that they already spend considerable extra time with women they suspect of being depressed. Many of those who have become used to routine screening report that this gives a structure to their work and added confidence in their ability to help mothers with depression. With regard to the second point, as Seeley (2001) remarked, 'the scale is only as good as the person using it. Where there is no, or inadequate training, individual health visitors will use it as best they can, but this may not be good enough'.

To screen or not to screen, to coin a phrase from our Australian colleagues, is a question currently being debated both in Britain and abroad. An extensive review in Australia (Buist *et al*, 2002) concluded that screening for antenatal and postnatal depression is likely to be useful because of the high prevalence of depressive disorders at both times and because of evidence that depression can be effectively treated. Early intervention may also have substantial benefits for the woman's partner, infant and older children. The researchers have argued that the case for screening outweighs that against, although they acknowledge that there are major challenges inherent in implementing such a programme and the need to evaluate outcome. A new research project, the National Postnatal Depression Prevention and Early Intervention

Programme, will evaluate outcomes of EPDS screening in terms of acceptability, cost-effectiveness, access and satisfaction, with management of up to 100 000 women in five states across Australia.

Many primary care trusts in the UK have already taken the screening initiative; a survey of EPDS screening practice carried out by the Scottish Intercollegiate Guidelines Network (SIGN; 2002) development group found that EPDS screening is undertaken routinely in all but one primary care trust area in Scotland. SIGN recommends the use of the EPDS as a screening tool, but the document also points out that:

'the routine use of the EPDS carries significant implications associated with ongoing training, health visitor time for screening and intervention, and facilities in general practice and secondary care for treatment' (p. 17).

Similar conclusions were reached in Sweden, where Sundelin & Håkansson (2000) reported that:

'Some Child Health Centres in the country are engaged in screening and treatment of postnatal depression, an activity which should be expanded. It is then required that adequate post-training is offered to the child health staff, and firm links established with general practitioners and psychiatrists. Before recommending general screening for postnatal depression, a screening trial should be implemented and evaluated in, for example, one county' (p. 77).

Although many health authorities in England have already introduced routine screening with the EPDS, this has recently been questioned by the National Screening Committee (NSC), which feels that there has been insufficient research into the use of the EPDS in clinical practice to justify a national initiative (see Coyle & Adams, 2002, for a fuller discussion of this issue). The NSC is calling for a large-scale community-based validation, which should include measures of cost-efficiency and the availability and effectiveness of referral pathways. We fully support this position and hope that national research committees will call for these studies to be undertaken.

The steering committee

Before starting a postnatal initiative, it is essential to set up an inter-disciplinary steering committee with representatives from maternity, obstetric and psychiatric primary care services. The committee should produce recommendations on services and guidelines consistent with the services available in the locality. All services should be informed of the new programme and of decisions reached by the committee.

A shared framework of understanding

The phrase 'postnatal depression' is often loosely used to describe a range of symptoms from tearfulness and emotional lability to the disconnection from reality of puerperal psychosis. Interpretation depends on both the user and the context. A psychiatrist, for example, may define a minor depression in very different terms from those used by a woman experiencing it. To avoid misunderstandings and ensure that each woman receives individualised care, it is important that all professionals have a shared understanding of the range of severity and possible origins of the condition and of various intervention options, including psychological measures as well as medication (Holden, 1996).

Health professionals' knowledge

When we first started our own research in 1983, we asked a general practitioner to give us the views of family doctors. We were rather surprised to learn that, in his opinion, most doctors knew little about postnatal depression, which was not at that time included in the training of undergraduates. Most doctors, he believed, learned about the condition only by being confronted with depressed women in their practice, and as we knew from our own previous research, the majority of mothers with depression remained undiagnosed.

Has this changed in the past two decades? Not according to recent research. Small and her colleagues in Australia compared the views held by 134 undergraduate medical students about postnatal depression with those of 60 women who had themselves experienced it (Small *et al*, 1997). The women's and students' views differed markedly: students were much more likely to view hormonal and biological factors and a 'tendency to depression' as being relevant, whereas the women tended to identify a wide range of social, physical health and life-event factors as contributing to their experience of depression. Fourth-year students tended to overestimate the prevalence of depression and sixth-year students to underestimate it. Both student groups underestimated the duration of depression compared with women's actual experiences. The authors concluded that medical students need to develop a broader understanding of maternal depression after the birth of a baby, and that women's own views of the experience can and should make an important contribution to medical teaching on this topic.

Aitken & Jacobson (1997), who sent a questionnaire to 173 psychiatrists and 350 general practitioners in the UK, found that these groups had a low level of awareness and knowledge of the EPDS, had little experience in its use and would not feel confident in giving advice on issues arising from its use by health visitors.

Our own counselling study (Holden *et al*, 1989) (see Chapter 4, this volume) and Boath *et al*'s (1999) comparison of routine treatment with treatment at a parent and baby day unit revealed differences in clinical outcome that clearly demonstrate the need to provide training to health professionals on how to detect and treat postnatal depression.

The role of nurses in postnatal depression

Mead *et al* (1997) examined the potential and current role and training needs of nurses. They found that although nurses are already involved in emotional health care with a variety of patient groups, this is not always acknowledged as mental health work. They explain that there is clear potential for an expanded role but little consensus regarding what role would be most effective for each nursing group, and few educational interventions have been demonstrated to be of proven effectiveness. With regard to counselling women with postnatal depression, Elliott (1994: p. 230) raised a pertinent question, asking 'Is this what health visitors should be doing?' As she pointed out, health visitors are not a treatment agency, although 'pressure of work often finds them operating a crisis intervention or treatment service.' Corney (1980), who studied referrals to social workers by health visitors, found that they rarely referred clients with emotional or relationship problems, but tried to help them by providing social support and making more-frequent visits, sometimes several times a week. In cases of depression, the health visitor would become someone the client could talk to, someone to be there when the client cries. They would often encourage clients to express their feelings, but were sometimes anxious that they would 'get out of their depth.'

The results of community-based intervention trials by a number of teams discussed in the previous chapter indicate strongly that if health visitors are given adequate training and support, they can positively influence the outcome for women in their care who have postnatal depression (Holden *et al*, 1989; Gerrard *et al*, 1994; Seeley *et al*, 1996; Wickberg & Hwang, 1996a; Cooper & Murray, 1997; Elliott *et al*, 2000). This has been confirmed in other trials in the UK: Taylor (1989), Angeli & Grahame (1990), Cullinan (1991) and Painter (1995) all reported that using the EPDS and supportive counselling led to increased identification and decreased symptoms among women with postnatal depression in their care and also increased the confidence of the health visitors in caring for them.

Not all countries have health visitors and there is a role for other nurses, including community psychiatric nurses, in postnatal depression. Studies in other countries have examined the ways in which primary care or hospital-based nurses can become involved with the evaluation of postnatal depression and the provisions of mother-oriented care. A few examples are Holt (1995, New Zealand) – EPDS identification by primary care nurses; Webster *et al* (2000, New Zealand) – midwives identifying postnatal depression and comparing the responses of European and Maori women; and Schaper *et al* (1994, Wisconsin, USA) – EPDS identification by midwives and doctors. Stamp & Crowther (1994, Australia) looked at mothers' perceptions of midwives' care and

attitudes, while Small *et al* (2000, Melbourne, Australia), who exami
the effectiveness of midwifery debriefing of postnatal women in
prevention of postnatal depression, found that, on the whole, this
unhelpful. Suzuki (2001, Japan), on the other hand, described a midw
led perinatal support system which emphasises the importance
ensuring that the views and feelings of women are acknowledged.

It seems clear that nurses are increasingly involved in caring for
emotional needs of their clients and, in particular, in finding ways
help women with postnatal depression. It is, however, important b
for the professionals and for the women they care for, that the poten
difficulties of such an extended role are clearly acknowledged and de
with by management.

Willingness and cooperation are not enough. Recognition of
extra time needed, standardised training programmes and assurar
that expert help and support from psychiatrists, psychologists a
community psychiatric nurses are readily accessible are essent
prerequisites for any postnatal depression programme to be successf

The need for clearly identified referral systems

Many cases of postnatal depression can be dealt with at primary ca
level with monitoring by the family doctor and brief interventions
primary care staff. However, most of those who will be administerir
the EPDS are unlikely to have in-depth psychiatric knowledge. Th
health visitor or primary care nurse should not be expected to take so
responsibility for deciding, on the basis of a raised EPDS score, who
depressed or who is suitable for an intervention. In the first instanc
decisions should be made in collaboration with the family doctor. (Se
Chapter 7 for an extended mood assessment interview.)

Many of those who cannot be helped by simple measures do not nee
expensive psychiatric assessments, but do need longer or more
specialist therapy. Some women will definitely require more-intensiv
help. Those caring for perinatal women need to know where and how t
refer, and they need to know that psychiatrists, psychologists and
community psychiatric nurses are not only willing and able to accep
referrals, but understand the special needs of this client group.

The need for specialist psychiatric services

In *The Confidential Enquiry into Maternal Deaths in the United Kingdom*,
Oates writes:

'there has been little improvement in the care for those suffering from severe
mental illness in association with childbirth. The majority of women who
suffer from these conditions still do not have access to mental health

specialist knowledge and skills, nor to a mother-and-baby
require admission for puerperal psychosis' (Oates, 2001:

secondary prevention of impact on the child and family,
natal period women should be seen more quickly than is
ical secondary care psychology or psychotherapy service.
has been decided that primary care staff will treat a
pression, problems may arise that are beyond the staff's
ledge. They are likely to encounter many ambiguous
ng for complex decisions; for example, a woman may
ry of personal abuse, suicidal impulses or fears that she
child. Referral policy should be clear and simple (see

eviously recommended that within each health district at
munity psychiatric nurses should be identified who have
esponsibility for the prevention and treatment of post-
disorder and can provide essential back-up to other health
(Cox, 1989). A specialist consultant psychiatrist would
propriate use of resources; Oates (1996) demonstrated that
istrict with 500 000 inhabitants, seeing all referred women
under 1 year of age would justify a full-time consultant

s of scores on item 10, self-harm

committee will need to decide on a policy with respect to
res on item 10 of the EPDS, which asks about self-harm.
en a worry to health professionals without mental health
ns who administer the scale. They need the reassurance of
lines, and the subject should be included in their training.
feelings are a fairly common symptom of depression. In tape-
iterviews conducted after the intervention in our counselling
of the women confessed to having felt desperate during
ession:

ad and unhappy and miserable before, but never to the extent that
Thomas, to the point where I just didn't want to live any more'.

t been for the wee one, I'd definitely have jumped' (Holden, 1988).

eassuring to know that the majority of women with a small
unlikely to act on such feelings. When Louis Appleby (1991)
tively examined population data from England and Wales for
1984, he found that the rate of suicide among women in the
tnatal year was only one-sixth of that expected in a matched
population. However, the Confidential Inquiry into Maternal

Deaths in the United Kingdom (Oates, 2001) found that, although rare (only 1 or 2 per 100 000 maternities), death from suicide is the most common cause of maternal deaths.

None of the women who died by suicide between 1997 and 1999 had been managed by a specialist perinatal mental health team, nor had any been admitted at any time to a mother-and-baby unit. Although a large number of the women were in contact with psychiatric or substance misuse services at the time of death, and eight were in-patients, there was a lack of information from psychiatric or social services in the documentation about their deaths (Oates, 2001: p. 185). The report also explains that the ICD–10 does not count such deaths as having a maternal cause, with the effect that not all such deaths were reported to the Oates inquiry, especially after the women had lost contact with community midwives. It was concluded that reporting mechanisms must be strengthened (p. 33).

There is as yet little published evidence linking suicidal ideation and risk with responses to item 10 on the EPDS. However, one interesting community-based study found that an indication of thoughts of self-harm on the EPDS did not necessarily alert health professionals. In Rochester, Minnesota, where universal screening was implemented in all community postnatal care sites, some degree of suicidal ideation was noted on the EPDS by 48 women, but this was acknowledged in the medical records of only 10 women, including one who required immediate hospitalisation (Georgiopoulos et al, 2001).

A positive score on item 10 should be taken seriously and action taken. This will usually involve an extra home visit to women whose EPDS score indicates more than the usual level of problems. The women screened, as well as health professionals, should be aware of what is involved in screening, and information for women should indicate that, if they need to speak to someone sooner, they should not hesitate to contact their health visitor or family doctor, or walk into the emergency clinic in a local psychiatric facility.

Training and support

There is a clear need for training for all health professionals in the nature, detection and treatment of perinatal depression, in understanding the experiences of the women, and in the development of listening skills and willingness to elicit and discuss psychological issues. For those implementing a postnatal depression service the training should also include the use of the EPDS and how to administer it sensitively. Training should also include awareness of the risk of suicide in depression, and, specifically, give guidelines on how to handle a positive response to item 10 on the EPDS.

Dealing with other people's emotional problems can be very taxing, especially if these resonate with the helper's own sadness or insecurities. The nature of this work is such that training should be followed by ongoing support and consultation from a mental health professional with counselling or therapy training, preferably one trained as a trainer for postnatal depression systems.

A range of prevention and intervention strategies should be explored, including individual and peer support, one-to-one counselling, antidepressants and the setting up of therapy or support groups in conjunction with mental health staff.

Counselling training

Health professionals who wish to add non-directive counselling to their repertoire of helping skills will need specific extra training and the acknowledgement of their managers that this extra service needs extra time. Not all health visitors will wish to become personally involved in counselling women with depression, and most family doctors would find counselling too time-consuming. Many primary care teams now have specialist counsellors working in the practice; alternatively, one member of the team could become a specialist in postnatal depression counselling.

Conclusions

It must be emphasised that the EPDS is merely a screen for depression that reveals dysphoria or low mood at the time of completion and indicates a need for further assessment. It does not provide a differential diagnosis of mental disorder, nor can it replace clinical judgement. Screening does not in itself constitute an intervention, nor, on its own, does it improve outcomes (Gilbody *et al*, 2001). Screening gives an indication of a women's need for help and should be a precursor to diagnosis and intervention.

Health professionals have told us that they become considerably involved with women they suspect of being depressed, but they are often unsure what to do. With adequate training, support and liaison with other services, it should be possible to develop a structured and effective approach to promoting the psychological well-being of women during the postnatal period. This could also help to maximise the time available to health professionals and, by providing a clear definition of their role, give increased confidence in their ability to offer constructive help to this important client group.

Using the Edinburgh Postnatal Depression Scale

This chapter summarises practical information for administering the Edinburgh Postnatal Depression Scale (EPDS; Cox *et al*, 1987), based on our own research experience and on feedback from health visitors in training.

How to use the EPDS

(1) Ask the woman to underline the response that comes closest to how she has felt during the previous 7 days.

(2) Ensure that all 10 items are completed.

(3) The woman should complete the EPDS herself, unless she has difficulty with reading, and she should not discuss her answers when completing the scale.

(4) The EPDS can be used routinely to screen for postnatal depression, or to provide further information before referral of a woman who seems to be depressed.

(5) EPDS items are scored from 0 to 3; the normal response scores 0 and the 'severe' response scores 3. Total the individual item scores (see the EPDS scoring sheet in Appendix 1).

(6) A total score of 12 or above was taken in the three-centre study (Gerrard *et al*, 1994) research as an indicator that the individual should be further assessed. Some authorities prefer a lower cut-off, to ensure that depressions are not missed (see Ahapter 2, this volume).

(7) Scores alone should not replace clinical judgement: women should be further assessed before deciding on treatment.

(8) Women who are already being treated for depression or other psychiatric problems would normally be excluded, unless they expressly wish to complete the scale.

Using the EPDS in research

As has already been discussed, the EPDS has been shown to be a useful way of accessing the emotional well-being of women in a given population. Research uses include:

- determining the percentage of women with low mood
- investigating the correlates of low mood
- in longitudinal studies, determining risk factors for low mood
- first-stage screening in epidemiological community studies
- first-stage screening to identify women with depression for an intervention trial
- monitoring changes over time in depressive symptoms in clinical intervention trials
- determining the need for intervention for postnatal depression.

A number of studies report that 'depression was measured using the EPDS'. This is incorrect: a single EPDS score above threshold does not indicate that an individual has depression, only that sufficient depressive symptoms are present to make this likely. If the EPDS is used as a stand-alone measure, then it can be claimed only that women did or did not have scores above the chosen threshold. For some studies this is acceptable. However, in studies in which it is important to know whether women are currently depressed (such as recruitment to an intervention trial, or measuring the success or otherwise of an intervention), the scale should be accompanied by a reliable clinical assessment interview.

Using the EPDS in clinical practice

Routine use of the EPDS has a number of advantages:

- it raises awareness of the possibility of postnatal depression among health professionals, women themselves and their families
- it may provide additional information when referring a woman to the general practitioner or to the perinatal mental health team
- it can provide the opportunity for early preventive intervention
- it gives women 'permission to speak' and health professionals 'permission to listen'
- it can help a woman to recognise and discuss her negative feelings
- it may change women's perception of what health professionals can offer
- it can provide a structured approach to identification of low mood or depression, clarifying the situation for both the woman and the professional
- it can be used to monitor progress in treatment
- it may help to prevent suicide
- it can lead to improved liaison with other professionals
- evidence of the number of high-scoring women may alert health authorities and management to the need for extra services, or redeployment of existing services.

The EPDS does not provide a differential diagnosis of mental disorder, nor can it replace clinical judgement. A high score does not necessarily imply that a woman has depression: she may simply be having a 'bad day', for example because of sleeplessness or temporary emotional or task overload. The opportunity to talk about her problems at a single interview may be sufficient to help her. Similarly, a low score does not always mean that a woman does not have depression: she may be unwilling or afraid to reveal her true feelings. One high score may indicate only that the woman is feeling temporarily overwhelmed by her circumstances or that she is tired and miserable on a particular day. Two high scores separated by 2 weeks, plus an interview, will usually confirm depression.

Honesty of women's responses

There is no mystery about the meaning of the EPDS items, and it would certainly not be difficult to obtain a deliberately high or low score. In fact, the highest-scoring woman in our counselling trial (Holden *et al*, 1989) was assesssed by the research psychiatrist as having a personality disorder: she enjoyed being the focus of attention. Health professionals have expressed particular concern about a total score of zero, especially if it seems that the woman is having problems: one would be very unlikely to obtain a zero score by answering honestly. However, as we have seen, the results of the EPDS validation studies (where an unseen EPDS score is compared with a diagnostic interview) indicate that most completed EPDS forms do accurately reflect the woman's feelings. If you are genuinely concerned, discuss the case with your line manager or the woman's family doctor.

What if someone does not wish to complete an EPDS?

There are many reasons why a woman may not wish to participate in screening. She may already be receiving treatment for depression; she may be currently depressed but afraid to reveal her feelings in case of possible repercussions (a health professional's concern for the infant, referral, fear of stigmatisation); or she may not be depressed and simply wishes to retain her privacy. Completing an EPDS is not compulsory. However, it does provide health professionals with an opportunity to identify women who may need help. The way the scale is presented is important, as is how the woman perceives that the information she reveals will be used. If a woman does not wish to avail herself of this opportunity, that is her absolute right and her wishes must be respected.

When, where and how should the EPDS be given?

Our original thinking (Cox *et al*, 1987) was that the EPDS could be given by health visitors during the postnatal check-up in the general practitioner's surgery or baby clinic at about 6 weeks, and this was done in our own research. In practice, we found that the 6-week EPDS picked up large numbers of women who, when interviewed by the research psychiatrist 4 to 6 weeks later, were not (or were no longer) depressed. Although it has been shown (e.g. Seeley *et al*, 1996; Cooper & Murray, 1997) that early interventions lead to improved outcome for both mothers and their infants, at 6 weeks postnatally many women are still adjusting to the birth, to sleeplessness and to the turmoil of having a new infant. A large number of high scores are likely to be obtained if the EPDS is given routinely in the very early weeks, which may lead to intervention overload for health professionals.

The EPDS may be given during antenatal or postnatal check-ups, immunisation or developmental screening. It is important that suitable accommodation and privacy are arranged so that women can complete the scale without feeling pressured, and that there is someone to 'hold the baby' during this process. There should be a secure box into which the completed forms may be posted, a fail-safe system of when and by whom they will be reviewed, and a clear policy of action to be taken for women who score above threshold. Remember, though, that mothers with depression are unlikely to be regular clinic attenders, so a home visit may be required for those who do not attend. If all else fails (and also for women who return to work early), the EPDS may be posted with an explanatory letter (and stamped addressed envelope for return), but again, bear in mind that non-responders may be depressed.

The argument for an EPDS home visit

It may be useful here to digress and describe how protocol in a particular area may be decided. In 1996, J. H. was asked to train 80 health visitors who would cascade the information to their colleagues as part of a postnatal depression initiative covering the whole of Glasgow. All Glasgow midwives also received a modified training. The steering committee included representatives of all health services who would be involved in the new programme, including psychiatrists, community psychiatric nurses, psychologists, family doctors, health visitors, midwives and obstetricians. There were also representatives of voluntary agencies in the Glasgow area. Decisions about the protocol for the new venture were reached only after extensive discussions over several weeks.

At this time, health visitors were a scarce resource in Glasgow and, their numbers having been recently considerably reduced, each had a very large case-load. They told me that they considered themselves lucky if they were able to pay one home visit to new mothers, after which, unless the women attended the well-baby clinic, she was unlikely to be seen again until the infant's hearing check-up at about 10 months after birth.

One important decision to be made for the protocol was the timing of the EPDS and where it should be administered. It was decided that, as the health visitors had to justify all their contacts, it would be given during an extra home visit to every new mother between 8 and 10 weeks postnatally. This gave the health visitors a contact time recognised by management and by the women themselves as being specifically for the mother. During this visit, the woman would complete the EPDS by herself, and then have the opportunity to talk about issues and feelings that may have been released. Both psychiatrists and comunity psychiatric nurses felt that this opportunity for discussion was important, particularly as it gave the health visitor the chance to make a preliminary on-the-spot assessment of the woman's mood. Indeed, some community psychiatric nurses felt that it would be unethical to administer an EPDS without the opportunity for feedback and further discussion of the woman's feelings, especially with women who scored above threshold.

Seeley (2001) found that this approach can be easily dovetailed into the routine feedback from the EPDS and using this approach enables an assessment of the mother's mood to be made.

Similar decision-making processes took place in NHS regions in Ireland and Scotland. The steering committees here also reached the conclusion that EPDS screening should be carried out during a designated home visit.

In answer to National Screening Committee concerns about screening with the EPDS discussed earlier, the Community Practitioners' and Health Visitors' Association (CPHVA) has issued guidelines for health visitors on using the EPDS as part of a maternal mood assessment. As these guidelines derived from a combined body of clinical experience and expertise and are thus of considerable importance to health visitors and to others using the EPDS in the UK and overseas, we reproduce them here in full:

'The CPHVA supports the view that the EPDS remains a very useful aid to professional judgement and a clinical interview for the detection of PND. Indeed, we are supported by the Scottish Intercollegiate Network Guidelines (2002) which state that the EPDS should be offered to women in the post-natal period as part of a screening programme for postnatal depression ... [F]ollowing extensive consultation the CPHVA would like to make the following recommendations for the use of the EPDS:

- The EPDS should never be used in isolation, it should form part of a full and systematic mood assessment of the mother, supporting professional judgement and a clinical interview.

- The EPDS should be only used by professionals who have been trained in the detection and management of PND, use of the EPDS and conducting a clinical interview.
- Formal mood assessments should only be carried out in a place where the mother is ensured privacy and when the professional has time to discuss the outcome and suitable interventions with the mother should they be necessary.
- The EPDS should never be used in an open clinic or posted to mothers. If the clinic is not busy and there are facilities to ensure privacy for the mother it may be the preferred option for some health visitors unable to do a home visit.
- Before using it the professional should consider possible factors which could influence the mother's comprehension of the purpose of the EPDS and her ability to complete the questions accurately, for example, literacy level, cultural background or language difficulties.
- Having asked the mother to complete the scale, the professional should discuss her individual responses one by one, being alert to a mismatch with her (or his) clinical impression, for example, mothers with puerperal psychosis may score low on the EPDS.
- Use of the EPDS should be followed by a clinical interview that utilises the nine symptoms from DSM–IV to ascertain depressive symptoms. Such an interview should also explore physical, emotional or social causes for the symptoms so that appropriate interventions can be discussed with the mother.

A specific score on the EPDS does not definitely confirm or refute the presence of PND. What it does offer is an indicator as to its possible presence, absence or severity. Is it reasonable, then, to consider whether much attention should be given to the score? The CPHVA believes that the score does have a quantitative value to the service provider, as when it is recorded it can support a needs assessment for service provision. It also serves as a benchmark for changes in the mother's mood or in response to a change in service. We believe that from the individual mother's viewpoint, while noting the score, the health visitor should rely on her fuller mood assessment to determine the severity of any depression. This is a qualitative approach and as such client-centred.' (Coyle & Adams, 2002: p. 395)

We regard this important policy statement by the CPHVA as consistent with the recommendations in this book. The debate initiated by the National Screening Committee is a potent spur to further develop the evidence base for a perinatal mental health service.

The CPHVA goes on to recommend the DSM–IV-based clinical interview, described by Seeley (2001), who trained the health visitors in the Cambridge study and has extensive knowledge of the use of the EPDS in practice. Seeley argues cogently for extra time to be spent with women when the EPDS is completed (presumably especially with those women who score above threshold), allowing at least 10 minutes for feedback from the EPDS and systematically augmenting it with DSM–IV criteria for depression. This involves going through the DSM–IV symptoms to tease out more of the woman's experience and the effect on her life, in particular the persistency and pervasiveness of the depressive symptoms. Again, we endorse this use of the EPDS.

Taking action on high scores

Any woman who scores above the chosen threshold should be given the opportunity for further discussion and assessment, usually within 2 weeks (follow local policy guidelines). Encourage her to talk about her responses to the EPDS items and about her feelings generally. If, on assessment, it seems clear that her low mood is temporary, reassure her that you and her family doctor are available for further help and let her know how to contact you if she feels the need.

A repeated high score 2 weeks later almost certainly indicates depression and the need for further assessment and intervention. A woman who has more than a transient low mood should be persuaded to see her doctor for assessment. A set number of extra weekly supportive listening visits may be offered by the health visitor and/or antidepressants may be prescribed by the family doctor. The woman should be reviewed using the EPDS after an appropriate time interval. Women who do not respond to these simple measures may need to see a psychologist or be referred for further psychiatric assessment.

See Chapter 6 for a discussion on what to do if an individual has any score on item 10 which indicates suicidal feelings.

Computerised EPDS

Computerised versions of the EPDS have been produced and validated by Glaze & Cox (1991). They reported that women were quite happy to complete the scale in this way. Computerisation reduces demand on staff time and permits introduction of the EPDS even when staffing levels are low. Among the disadvantages of the computerised EPDS are that staff might require training in the use of the computer, that data protection needs special attention and that, unless laptop computers are provided, administration would be restricted to one setting (so that mothers with depression, who are often unwilling to leave their homes, would be missed (Elliott, 1994)).

Antenatal use

The EPDS may also be used in pregnancy, either routinely or to identify suspected depressions. In our three-centre training study, we asked health visitors to give an EPDS to every woman at about 28 weeks antenatally, both to introduce the idea that health professionals are concerned with women's emotional well-being and to detect depression. In Murray & Cox's (1990) validation of the EPDS in pregnancy, midwives screened all pregnant women, as they did in the Cambridge prenatal study (Green, 1998) and in the Avon study, reported by Evans *et al* (2001). As Evans *et al* point out, however, the benefits of routine antenatal screening have not yet been demonstrated by research.

Who should give the EPDS?

Although our research in UK has concentrated on the use of the EPDS by health visitors and midwives, it can be administered by any health professional who understands its use, including doctors, psychologists, midwives and community psychiatric nurses. Irrespective of who administers the scale, the importance of a team approach to intervention cannot be overemphasised.

Record-keeping

Where to keep completed EPDS forms should be a management decision, but as a general rule, information about the mother should always be kept with her own health records, not with those of the infant. Remember that this material is strictly confidential. It should not be divulged to anyone outside the health care team without the woman's knowledge and consent.

Using the EPDS with non-English speakers

A translation of the EPDS or the English-language version explained by an interpreter may be used to open the subject for discussion, but only a validated translation may be assumed to give scores that have the same meaning as those from the original English. Cultural differences in interpretation might result in a score that does not accurately reflect the mother's mood (see Chapter 3).

Conclusions

Routine use of the EPDS in health care settings may prevent much suffering, by identifying women who need treatment and reassuring those whose low mood is temporary. It might also help to persuade women that it is safe to talk about negative feelings. However, EPDS screening should be carried out only by health care professionals with an understanding of postnatal depression who have been specifically trained in its use. It should be given in the context of a confidential interview, preferably in the woman's own home, and it should be followed up when necessary by a clinical assessment.

The Edinburgh Postnatal Depression Scale

How are you feeling?

As you have recently had a baby, we would like to know how you are feeling now. Please <u>underline</u> the answer which comes closest to how you have felt in the past 7 days, not just how you feel today. Here is an example, already completed:

I have felt happy:
Yes, most of the time
<u>Yes, some of the time</u>
No, not very often
No, not at all

This would mean: 'I have felt happy some of the time during the past week'. Please complete the other questions in the same way.

In the past 7 days

1. I have been able to laugh and see the funny side of things:
   As much as I always could
   Not quite so much now
   Definitely not so much now
   Not at all

2. I have looked forward with enjoyment to things:
   As much as I ever did
   Rather less than I used to
   Definitely less than I used to
   Hardly at all

3. I have blamed myself unnecessarily when things went wrong:
   Yes, most of the time
   Yes, some of the time
   Not very often
   No, never

---

4. I have been anxious or worried for no good reason:
   No, not at all
   Hardly ever
   Yes, sometimes
   Yes, very often

5. I have felt scared or panicky for no very good reason:
   Yes, quite a lot
   Yes, sometimes
   No, not much
   No, not at all

6. Things have been getting on top of me:
   Yes, most of the time I haven't been able to cope at all
   Yes, sometimes I haven't been coping as well as usual
   No, most of the time I have coped quite well
   No, I have been coping as well as ever

7. I have been so unhappy that I have had difficulty sleeping:
   Yes, most of the time
   Yes, sometimes
   Not very often
   No, not at all

8. I have felt sad or miserable:
   Yes, most of the time
   Yes, quite often
   Not very often
   No, not at all

9. I have been so unhappy that I have been crying:
   Yes, most of the time
   Yes, quite often
   Only occasionally
   No, never

10. The thought of harming myself has occurred to me:
    Yes, quite often
    Sometimes
    Hardly ever
    Never

Edinburgh Postnatal Depression Scale: scoring sheet

1. I have been able to laugh and see the funny side of things:
   As much as I always could   0
   Not quite so much now   1
   Definitely not so much now   2
   Not at all   3

2. I have looked forward with enjoyment to things:
   As much as I ever did   0
   Rather less than I used to   1
   Definitely less than I used to   2
   Hardly at all   3

3. I have blamed myself unnecessarily when things went wrong:
   Yes, most of the time   3
   Yes, some of the time   2
   Not very often   1
   No, never   0

4. I have been anxious or worried for no good reason:
   No, not at all   0
   Hardly ever   1
   Yes, sometimes   2
   Yes, very often   3

5. I have felt scared or panicky for no very good reason:
   Yes, quite a lot   3
   Yes, sometimes   2
   No, not much   1
   No, not at all   0

6. Things have been getting on top of me:
   Yes, most of the time I haven't been able to cope at all   3
   Yes, sometimes I haven't been coping as well as usual   2
   No, most of the time I have coped quite well   1
   No, I have been coping as well as ever   0

7. I have been so unhappy that I have had difficulty sleeping:
   Yes, most of the time   3
   Yes, sometimes   2
   Not very often   1
   No, not at all   0

8. I have felt sad or miserable:
    Yes, most of the time 3
    Yes, quite often 2
    Not very often 1
    No, not at all 0

9. I have been so unhappy that I have been crying:
    Yes, most of the time 3
    Yes, quite often 2
    Only occasionally 1
    No, never 0

10. The thought of harming myself has occurred to me:
    Yes, quite often 3
    Sometimes 2
    Hardly ever 1
    Never 0

Translations of the Edinburgh Postnatal Depression Scale

The English-language Edinburgh Postnatal Depression Scale (EPDS) has been widely translated: this Appendix reproduces 20 of these translations. Key references, including validation studies where applicable, are given for each translation. The authors and publishers cannot vouch for the validity of any translations that have not undergone a positive validation, and would be grateful for any additional information on validation studies using these translations. Please contact the publishers if you wish to translate the EPDS into any language not listed below.

- Arabic (this unvalidated version appears with permission of the Pædiatric Mental Mental Health Service, SWSAHS, Liverpool, Australia)
- Chinese (Mandarin) (Lee *et al*, 1998)
- Czech (Dragonas *et al*, 1996)
- Dutch (Pop *et al*, 1992)
- French (Guedeney & Fermanian, 1998)
- German (Bergant *et al*, 1998; Muzik *et al*, 2000)
- Greek (Thorpe *et al*, 1992)
- Hebrew (Fisch *et al*, 1997; Glasser & Barell, 1999)
- Hindi (source not known)
- Icelandic (Thome, 1992, 1996, 1999)
- Japanese (Okano *et al*, 1996, 1998)
- Maltese (Felice, 1998)
- Norwegian (Eberhard-Gran *et al*, 2001)
- Portuguese (Areias *et al*, 1996a,b; Da-Silva *et al*, 1998)
- Punjabi (Clifford *et al*, 1997, 1999)
- Slovenian (M. Blinc Pesek, personal communication, 2003)
- Spanish (Jadresic *et al*, 1995; Vega-Dienstmaier *et al*, 2002)
- Swedish (Lundh & Gyllang, 1993; Wickberg & Hwang, 1996*b*)
- Urdu (source not known)
- Vietnamese (Matthey *et al*, 1997)

A full list of the translations of which we are aware is given in Chapter 3.

Arabic

سيدتي،

الرجاء أن تضعي خطاً تحت الجواب الذي يعبر بطريقة أدق عن كيفية شعورك في الأيام السبعة الماضية، وليس عن شعورك اليوم فحسب.

اليك مثل وقد أكمل

لقد شعرت باتني سعيدة
نعم كل الأوقات
نعم معظم الأوقات
كلا ليس في أحوال كثيرة
كلا أبداً

وهذا يعني: لقد شعرت باتني سعيدة معظم الوقت خلال الاسبوع الماضي. الرجاء أن تكملي الأسئلة الأخرى بالطريقة ذاتها.

نرجو أن تضعي خطاً تحت أحد الأجوبة التالية

خلال الأيام السبعة الماضية

١- لقد استطعت الشعور بالفرح والسعادة
- بالمقدار نفسه الذي استطعته قبلاً
- ليس تماماً بالمقدار نفسه الآن
- قطعاً ليس بالمقدار نفسه الآن
- كلا مطلقاً

٢- لقد تطلعت الى الأمور بتمتع
- بالمقدار نفسه مثل أي وقت مضى
- أقل نوعاً ما مما اعتدته
- قطعاً أقل مما اعتدته
- نادراً. أبداً

٣- لقد لمت نفسي بدون لزوم عندما سارت الأمور على غير ما يرام
- نعم في معظم الأحيان
- نعم في بعض الأحيان
- ليس في أحوال كثيرة
- كلا أبداً

٤- لقد كنت قلقة ومشغولة البال بدون سبب وجيه
  - كلا أبداً
  - نادراً
  - نعم في بعض الأحيان
  - نعم في أحوال كثيرة

٥- لقد شعرت بالخوف والذعر بدون سبب وجيه
  - نعم أكثر الأحيان
  - نعم في بعض الأحيان
  - كلا ليس كثيراً
  - كلا مطلقاً

٦- تراكمت الأعمال عليّ فلم استطع القيام بها كلها
  - نعم في معظم الأحيان لم استطع أبداً القيام بها
  - نعم في بعض الأحيان لم استطع القيام بها كالمعتاد
  - كلا لقد استطعت القيام بها في بعض الأحيان
  - كلا لقد استطعت القيام بها كالمعتاد

٧- لقد كنت غير سعيدة لدرجة انه كانت لديّ صعوبة في النوم
  - نعم في معظم الأحيان
  - نعم في بعض الأحيان
  - ليس كثيراً
  - كلا أبداً

٨- لقد شعرت بانني لست سعيدة وبائسة
  - نعم في معظم الأحيان
  - نعم أكثر الأحيان
  - كلا ليس أكثر الأحيان
  - كلا مطلقاً

٩- لقد كنت غير سعيدة وأشعر بألم مرير لدرجة كنت أبكي
  - نعم في معظم الأحيان
  - نعم أكثر الأحيان
  - فقط من وقت الى آخر
  - كلا أبداً

١٠- لقد خطرت لي فكرة الحاق الأذى بنفسي
  - نعم في أحوال كثيرة
  - نعم في بعض الأحيان
  - نادراً
  - كلا مطلقاً

Chinese (Mandarin)

得分

愛丁堡產後抑鬱量表(HK-EPDS2.0a)

姓名 _____ 年齡 _____ 新生孩子周歲 _____ 填表日期 _____

說明：因為您剛生了孩子，我們想了解一下您的感受。請選擇一個最能反映您過去七天感受的答案。

注意：不只是您今天的感覺，而是過去七天的感受。例如：

我感到愉快。 （1）所有時候這樣。

（2）大部分時候這樣。

（3）不經常這樣。

（4）一點也沒有。

選擇答案（2）表明在上一周內你大部分時間都感到愉快。請照同樣方法完成以下各題。

在過去七天內：

我能看到事物有趣的一面，並笑得開心。

（1） 同以前一樣。

（2） 沒有以前那麼多。

（3） 肯定比以前少。

（4） 完全不能。

2. 我欣然期待未來的一切。

（1） 同以前一樣。

（2） 沒有以前那麼多。

（3） 肯定比以前少。

（4） 完全不能。

3. 當事情出錯時，我會不必要地責備自己。

（1） 大部分時候這樣。

（2） 有時候這樣。

（3） 不經常這樣。

（4） 沒有這樣。

4. 我無緣無故感到焦慮和擔心。

（1） 一點也沒有。

（2） 極少有。

（3） 有時候這樣。

（4） 經常這樣。

5. 我無緣無故感到害怕和驚慌。

（1） 相當多時候這樣。

（2） 有時候這樣。

（3） 不經常這樣。

（4） 一點也沒有。

6. 很多事情衝著我而來，使我透不過氣。

（1） 大多數時候我都不能應付。

（2） 有時候我不能像平時那樣應付得好。

（3） 大部分時候我都能像平時那樣應付得好。

（4） 我一直都能應付得好。

7. 我很不開心，以致失眠。

（1） 大部分時候這樣。

（2） 有時候這樣。

（3） 不經常這樣。

（4） 一點也沒有。

8. 我感到難過和悲傷。

（1） 大部分時候這樣。

（2） 相當時候這樣。

（3） 不經常這樣。

（4） 一點也沒有。

9. 我不開心到哭。

（1） 大部分時候這樣。

（2） 有時候這樣。

（3） 只是間中這樣。

（4） 沒有這樣。

10. 我想過要傷害自己。

（1） 相當多時候這樣。

（2） 有時候這樣。

（3） 很少這樣。

（4） 沒有這樣。

Czech

Vaše pocity v minulém týdnu:

1. Byla jste schopna se smát a vidět věci i z veselé stránky:
   stejně jako dříve
   ne tak často jako dříve
   rozhodně ne tak často jako dříve
   vůbec ne

2. S radostí jsem se těšila na příští věci:
   stejně jako dříve
   poněkud méně mež dříve
   rozhodně méně než dřív
   skoro vůbec ne

3. Zbybečně jsem si vyčítala, když se něco nedařilo:
   ano, většinou
   ano, někdy
   ne moc často
   ne, nikdy

4. Cítila jsem úzkost nebo měla starosti bez přiměřeného důvodu:
   ne, vůbec ne
   skoro vůbec ne
   ano, někdy
   ano, často

5. Měla jsem strach nebo pocit paniky bez podstatného důvodu:
   ano, hodně
   ano, někdy
   ne, moc ne
   ne, vůbec ne

6. Věci mi přerůstaly přes hlavu, nestačila jsem:
   ano, většinou
   ano, někdy
   zcela výjimečně
   ne, vůbec ne

7. Byla jsem tak nešťastná, že jsem měla potíže se spánkem:
   ano, většinou
   někdy
   ne moc často
   ne, vůbec ne

8. Bylo mi smutno nebo mizerně:
   ano, většinou
   ano, dost často
   ne moc často
   ne, vůbec ne

9. Byla jsem tak nešťastná, že jsem plakala:
   ano, většinou
   ano, dost často
   jen sřídka
   ne, nikdy

10. Naspadaly mne myělvenky, že si něco udělám:
    ano, dost často
    někdy
    sotvakdy
    nikdy

Dutch

De volgende vragen hebben betrekking up hoe u zich de afgelopen 7 dagen heeft gevoeld. Kruis dat antwoord aan dat het beste aangeeft hoe u zich voelde.

1. Ik heb kunnen lachen en de zonnige kant van de dingen kunnen inzien:
   Zoveel als ik altijd kon
   Niet zo veel nu als anders
   Zeker niet zo veel nu als anders
   Helemaal niet

2. Ik heb met plezier naar dingen uitgekeken:
   Zoals altijd of meer
   Wat minder dan ik gewend was
   Absoluut minder dan ik gewend was
   Nauwelijks

3. Ik heb mij zelf onnodig verwijten gemaakt als er iets fout ging:
   Ja, heel vaak
   Ja, soms
   Niet erg vaak
   Nee, nooit

4. Ik ben bang of bezorgd geweest zonder dat er een aanleiding was:
   Nee, helemaal niet
   Nauwelijks
   Ja, soms
   Ja, zeer vaak

5. Ik reageerde schrikachtig of paniekerig zonder echte goede reden:
   Ja, tamelijk vaak
   Ja, soms
   Nee, niet vaak
   Nooit

6. De dingen groeiden me boven het hoofd:
   Ja, meestal was ik er niet tegen opgewassen
   Ja, soms was ik minder goed tegen dingen opgewassen dan anders
   Nee, meestal kon ik de dingen erg goed aan
   Nee, ik kon alles even goed aan als anders

7. Ik voelde me zo ongelukkig dat ik er bijna niet van kon slapen:
   Ja, meestal
   Ja, soms
   Niet vaak
   Helemaal niet

8. Ik voelde me somber en beroerd:
   Ja, bijna steeds
   Ja, tamelijk vaak
   Niet erg vaak
   Nee, helemaal niet

9. Ik was zo ongelukkig dat ik heb zitten huilen:
   Ja, heel vaak
   Ja, tamelijk vaak
   Alleen af en toe
   Nee, nooit

10. Ik heb er aan gedacht om mezelf iets aan te doen:
    Ja, tamelijk vaak
    Soms
    Nauwelijks
    Nooit

French

Vous venez d'avoir un bébé. Nous aimerions savoir comment vous vous sentez. Nous vous demandons de bien vouloir remplir ce questionnaire en soulignant la réponse qui vous semble le mieux décrire comment vous vous êtes sentie durant la semaine (c'est-à-dire sur les 7 jours qui viennent de s'écouler) et pas seulement au jour d'aujourd'hui.

Voici un exemple

Je me suis sentie heureuse:
    Oui, tout le temps
    <u>Oui, la plupart du temps</u>
    Non, pas très souvent
    Non, pas du tout.

Ceci signifiera "je me suis sentie heureuse la plupart du temps durant la semaine qui vient de s'écouler". Merci de bien vouloir répondre aux autres questions.

PENDANT LA SEMAINE QUI VIENT DE S'ECOULER

1. J'ai pu rire et prendre les choses du bon côté:
    Aussi souvent que d'habitude
    Pas tout-à-fait autant
    Vraiment beaucoup moins souvent ces jours-ci
    Absolument pas

2. Je me suis sentie confiante et joyeuse, en pensant à l'avenir:
    Autant que d'habitude
    Plutôt moins que d'habitude
    Vraiment moins que d'habitude
    Pratiquement pas

3. Je me suis reprochée, sans raisons, d'être responsable quand les choses allaient mal:
    Oui, la plupart du temps
    Oui, parfois
    Pas très souvent
    Non, jamais

4. Je me suis sentie inquiète ou soucieuse sans motifs:
    Non, pas du tout
    Presque jamais
    Oui, parfois
    Oui, très souvent

5. Je me suis sentie effrayée ou paniquée sans vraiment de raisons:
   Oui, vraiment souvent
   Oui, parfois
   Non, pas très souvent
   Non, pas du tout

6. J'ai eu tendance à me sentir dépassée par les évènements:
   Oui, la plupart du temps, je me suis sentie incapable de faire face aux situations
   Oui, parfois, je ne me suis pas sentie aussi capable de faire face que d'habitude
   Non, j'ai pu faire face à la plupart des situations
   Non, je me suis sentie aussi efficace que d'habitude

7. Je me suis sentie si malheureuse que j'ai eu des problèmes de sommeil:
   Oui, la plupart du temps
   Oui, parfois
   Pas très souvent
   Non, pas du tout

8. Je me suis sentie triste ou peu heureuse:
   Oui, la plupart du temps
   Oui, très souvent
   Pas très souvent
   Non, pas du tout

9. Je me suis sentie si malheureuse que j'en ai pleuré:
   Oui, la plupart du temps
   Oui, très souvent
   Seulement de temps en temps
   Non, jamais

10. Il m'est arrivé de penser à me faire du mal:
   Oui, très souvent
   Parfois
   Presque jamais
   Jamais

German

Nachdem Sie kürzlich ein Baby hatten, würden wir gerne wissen, wie Sie sich fühlen.

Bitte, unterstreichen Sie die Antwort, die am ähnlichsten beschreibt, wie Sie sich in den letzten sieben Tagen gefühlt haben, nicht nur wie Sie sich heute fühlen:

Hier ist ein bereits ausgefülltes Beispiel:

Ich war glücklich:
- Ja, die ganze Zeit
- <u>Ja, meistens</u>
- Nein, nicht sehr oft
- Nein, gar nicht

Das würde bedeuten: "Ich habe mich den größten Teil der Zeit glücklich gefühlt, während dieser Woche." Bitte unterstreichen Sie die für Sie zutreffenden Antworten in derselben Weise.

IN DEN LETZTEN SIEBEN TAGEN

1. Ich konnte lachen und die komische Seite von Dingen sehen:
   - So viel wie bisher
   - Nicht ganz wie früher
   - Entschieden nicht so sehr wie bisher
   - Überhaupt nicht

2. Ich habe mich auf Dinge im Voraus gefreut:
   - So viel wie bisher
   - Wohl weniger als gewöhnlich
   - Entschieden weniger wie bisher
   - Kaum mehr

3. Ich habe mich unnötiger Weise schuldig gefühlt, wenn Dinge schief gingen:
   - Ja, meistens
   - Ja, gelegentlich
   - Nicht sehr oft
   - Nein, niemals

4. Ich war ängstlich oder besorgt ohne guten Grund:
   - Nein, gar nicht
   - Kaum
   - Ja, gelegentlich
   - Ja, sehr oft

5. Ich habe mich gefürchtet oder war in Panik ohne guten Grund:
   Ja, sehr häufig
   Ja, gelegentlich
   Nein, nicht viel
   Nein, überhaupt nicht

6. Dinge wurden mir zuviel:
   Ja, meistens konnte ich die Situation nicht meistern
   Ja, gelegentlich konnte ich die Dinge nicht so gut meistern wie sonst
   Nein, meistens konnte ich die Situation meistern
   Nein, ich bewältige Dinge so gut wie immer

7. Ich war so unglücklich, daß ich nur schlecht schlafen konnte:
   Ja, meistens
   Ja, gelegentlich
   Nein, nicht sehr häufig
   Nein, gar nicht

8. Ich habe mich traurig oder elend gefühlt:
   Ja, meistens
   Ja, gelegentlich
   Nein, nicht sehr häufig
   Nein, gar nicht

9. Ich war so unglücklich, daß ich weinte:
   Ja, den größten Teil der Zeit
   Ja, sehr häufig
   Nur gelegentlich
   Nein, nie

10. Der Gedanke, mir etwas anzutun, ist mir gekommen:
    Ja, recht häufig
    Gelegentlich
    Kaum jemals
    Niemals

Greek

1. Μπορούσα να γελώ και να βλέπω την αστεια πλευρά της ζωής:
   όπως πριν
   λιγότερο από πριν
   πολύ λιγότερο από πριν
   καθόλου

2. Εβλεπα το αύριο με ενθοθσιασμο:
   όπως και πριν
   μάλλον λιγότερο από πριν
   πολύ λιγότερο από πριν
   καθόλου

3. Κατηγορούσα άδικα τον εαυτό μου, χωρις να χρειάςεται, λια πράγματα που πηγαυ στραβά:
   ναι, όλη την ώρα
   ναι, αρκετά συχνά
   όχι πολύ συχνά
   ποτέ

4. Ενιωθα άγχος ή οτευοχώρια χωρις σοβαρό λόγο:
   όχι, καθόλου
   σχεδόν ποτέ
   ναι, καμιά φορά
   ναι, συχνά

5. ΕνιωΘα φόβο ή πανικο χωρις, σοβαρό λόγο:
   ναι, πολύ συχνα
   ναι, καμιά φορά
   όχι, όχι συχνά
   όχι, καθόλου

Την περασμένη εβδομάδα

6. Με πήρε η κάτω βόλτα (ένιωθα πολύ πεσμέυη):
   ναι, σχεδόν συνέχεια
   ναι, καμιά φορά
   όχι, σχεδόν ποτέ
   όχι, καθόλου

7. Ημουν τόσο στενοχωρημένη που δεν μπορούσα να κοιμηθώ:
   ναι, σχεδόν συνέχεια
   ναι, καμιά φορά
   πολύ σπάνια
   όχι, καθόλου

8. Ενιωθα θλιμένη ή πως ήμουν για λύπηση:
   ναι, σχεδόν συνέχεια
   ναι, αρκετά συχνά
   όχι, πολύ συχνά
   όχι, καθόλου

9. Ενιωθα τόσο δυστυχισμένη που έκλαιγα:
   ναι, όλη την ώρα
   ναι, αρκετά συχνά
   κάπου-κάπου
   όχι, ποτέ

10. Μου ήρθε να βλάψω τον εαυτό μού:
    ναι, αρκετά συχνά
    καμιά φορά
    σχεδόν ποτέ
    ποτέ

Hebrew

<u>הוראות למשתמש/ת:</u>

❖ היולדת מתבקשת לסמן את התשובה אשר מתאר בצורה הטובה ביותר את הרגשותיה בשבוע האחרון.

❖ חשוב שתענה על כל עשר השאלות.

❖ במידה שהיולדת לא ממלאת את השאלון בנוכחותך, חשוב להיזהר שהיא לא תדון על תשובותיה עם אדם אחר.

❖ רצוי שהיולדת תמלא את השאלון ללא עזרתך, אלא אם היא מתקשה בקריאה.

❖ ה-EPDS מתאים לשימוש במראה או בבית הנבדקת

• •

<u>השאלון:</u>

נא לסמן ליד משפט <u>אחד</u> בכל קבוצה את זה שמתאר בצורה הטובה ביותר את הרגשותיך <u>בשבוע האחרון</u>, כולל היום.

1. במשך השבוע האחרון, הייתי מסוגלת לצחוק ולראות את הצד המצחיק של דברים

____ כפי שיכולתי תמיד
____ פחות מתמיד
____ הרבה פחות מתמיד
____ בכלל לא

2. במשך השבוע האחרון, ציפיתי בהנאה לדברים שיקרו

____ כפי שיכולתי תמיד
____ פחות שהייתי רגילה
____ הרבה פחות משהייתי יכולה
____ כמעט בכלל לא

3.* במשך השבוע האחרון, האשמתי את עצמי שלא לצורך כאשר דברים לא הסתדרו

____כן, רוב הזמן
____כן, חלק מהזמן
____לעתים רחוקות
____אף פעם

4. במשך השבוע האחרון, הרגשתי חרדה או דאגה ללא כל סיבה

____בכלל לא
____לעתים רחוקות
____כן, לפעמים
____כן, לעתים קרובות מאד

5\.* במשך השבוע האחרון, הרגשתי מפוחדת או מבוהלת ללא כל סיבה מוצדקת

____כן, לעתים קרובות
____כן, לפעמים
____לעתים רחוקות
____בכלל לא

6\.* במשך השבוע האחרון, הרגשתי שהדברים קשים לי מדי

____כן, לרוב לא יכולתי להתמודד בכלל
____כן, לפעמים לא יכולתי להתמודד כפי שאני רגילה
____לא, בדרך כלל התמודדתי (הסתדרתי) די טוב
____לא, אני מתמודדת כמו תמיד

7\.* במשך השבוע האחרון, הרגשתי כה אומללה שהיה לי קשה לישון

____כן, בדרך כלל
____כן, לפעמים
____לעתים רחוקות
____בכלל לא

8\.* במשך השבוע האחרון, הרגשתי עצובה או אומללה (מצוברחת)

____כן, רוב הזמן
____כן, לעתים קרובות
____לעתים רחוקות
____בכלל לא

9\.* במשך השבוע האחרון, הרגשתי כה אומללה שבכיתי

____רוב הזמן
____לעתים קרובות
____רק מדי פעם
____בכלל לא

10\.* במשך השבוע האחרון, המחשבה לפגוע בעצמי עלתה בראשי

____כן, לעתים קרובות
____לפעמים
____כמעט ולא
____בכלל לא

ציונים: התשובות מקודדות 0, 1, 2, או 3, לפי חומרת התגובה. שאלות המסומנות ב*\ מקודדים הצורה הפוכה (3, 2, 1, 0). הציון הכולל נחשב ע"י סכום הציונים של כל השאלות.

הערות:

❖ למשתמשים ניתנת הרשות לשכפל את המבחן ללא אישור נוסף, בתנאי שמצוטטים את המקורות האוריגינלי והנוכחי על גבי כל טופס.

❖ שאלון ה-EPDS תורגם גם לשפה הרוסית וניתן לקבל גירסה זו מהמחברים.

Hindi

'आप कैसा महसूस कर रहीं हैं'

आपके यहां कुछ दिनों पहले बच्चे का जन्म हुआ है, हम यह जानना चाहते हैं कि अब आप कैसा महसूस कर रही हैं। पिछले एक हफ़्ते के दौरान में आपनें जैसा महसूस किया है, उसके सामने निशान (✓) लगा दें, न कि जैसा आप आज महसूस कर रही हैं।

यहाँ हल किया हुआ एक उदाहरण दे रहे हैं

मैने खुश महसूस किया है

हाँ, अधिकांश समय,

हाँ, कुछ समय ✓

नहीं, अकसर नहीं

नहीं, कभी नहीं

इसका मतलब है कि मैंने कुछ समय खुश महसूस किया है, पिछले एक हफ़्ते के दौरान । कृपया बाकि प्रश्नों का जबाब इसी तरह दें।

पिछले सात दिनों के दौरान'

1. मैं हंस पायी हूँ और बातों का अच्छा पहलू देख पायी हूँ:

जितना में सदैव करती पायी हूँ

अब उतना नहीं

निश्चित ही अब कम

बिल्कुल नहीं

2. मैं आने वाली बातों के प्रति खुशी महसूस करती हूँ

जितना में पहले कर पायी

जितना पहले कर पाती थी उससे कम

निश्चित रुप से पहले से कम

बिलकुल नहीं के बराबर

3. कुछ भी बिगड़ जाने पर में अनावश्यक रूप से अपने को दोषी मानती हूँ।

हाँ, अधिकांश समय

हाँ, कुछ समय

अकसर नहीं

नहीं बिलकुल नहीं

4. पर्याप्त कारण न होने पर भी मैं घबराई या चिंतित महसूस करती रही हूँ:

नहीं बिलकुल नहीं

शायद ही कभी

हाँ, कभी कभी

हाँ, अकसर ही

5. पर्याप्त कारण न होने पर भी मैं भयभीत या अत्याधिक घबराहट महसूस करती रही हूँ:

हाँ, काफी ज्यादा

हाँ, कभी कभी

नहीं, अधिक नहीं

नहीं, कभी नहीं

6. काम मुझे अपने ऊपर बोझ मालूम पड़ता रहा है:

हाँ, अधिकांश समय में झेल नहीं पायी हूँ

हाँ, कभी कभी में पहले की तरह झेल नहीं पायी हूँ

नहीं अधिकांश समय में अच्छे से झेल पायी हूँ

नहीं, मैं हमेशा की तरह ही झेल पायी हूँ

7. मैं इतना उदास महसूस करती रही हूँ कि मुझे नींद आने में परेशानी हुई :

हाँ, अधिकांश समय

हाँ, कभी कभी

अकसर नहीं

नहीं, बिलकुल नहीं

8. मैं उदास या दुखी महसूस करती हूँ:

हाँ, अधिकांश समय

हाँ, अकसर ही

अकसर नहीं

नहीं, कभी नहीं

9. मैं इतना दुखी रही हूँ कि रोती रही हूँ:

हाँ, अधिकांश समय

हाँ, अकसर ही

केवल, कभी कभी

नहीं, कभी नहीं

10. अपने आप को नुकसान/आत्म हत्या/ पहुंचाने का ख्याल मुझे आया है:

हाँ, अकसर ही

कभी, कभी

शायद ही कभी,

कभी नहीं

Icelandic

Með eftirfarandi spurningalista er verið að kanna líðan kvenna eftir barnsborð.
Vinsamlegast krossaðu framan við það svar sem kemst næst því að lýsa hvernig þér hefur liðið síðastliðna viku.

Mér hefur liðið þannig síðastliðna viku:

1. Ég hef getað hlegið og séð broslegu hliðarnar á lífinu
   Eins mikið og áður
   Ekki alveg eins mikið og áður
   Alls ekki eins mikið og áður
   Alls ekki

2. Ég hlakkaði til ýmissa atburða
   Alveg eins mikið og áður
   Aðeins minna en áður
   Mun minna en áður
   Varla nokkurn tímann

3. Ég hef ásakað sjálfa mig að ósekju þegar eitthvað fór úrskeiðis
   Já, yfirleitt
   Já, stundum
   Sjaldan
   Nei, aldrei

4. Ég hef verið kvíðin og áhyggjufull þó ég hafi ekki haft ástæðu til
   Nei, alls ekki
   Næstum aldrei
   Já, stundum
   Já, mjög oft

5. Ég hef verið hrædd eða strekkt á taugum þó ég hafi ekki haft ástæðu til
   Já, nokkuð oft
   Já, stundum
   Nei, sjaldan
   Nei, aldrei

6. Allt hefur vaxið mér yfir höfuð
   Já, oftast hef ég ekki getað ráðið við neitt
   Já, stundum hefur mér gengið verr en vanalega
   Nei, yfirleitt hefur allt gengið vel
   Nei, ég hef ráðið við hlutina eins og venjulega

7. Ég hef verið svo vansæl að ég hef átt erfitt með svefn
   Já, yfirleitt
   Já, stundum
   Sjaldan
   Nei, alls ekki

8. Ég hef verið döpur og aum
   Já, nær alltaf
   Já, frekar oft
   Sjaldan
   Nei, alls ekki

9. Ég hef verið svo vansæl að ég hef grátið
   Já, mjög oft
   Já, stundum
   Einstaka sinnum
           Nei, aldrei

10. Mér hefur dottið í hug að gera sjálfri mér mein
    Já, nokkuð oft
    Stundum
    Nær aldrei
    Aldrei

Japanese

エ ジ ン バ ラ 産 後 う つ 病 調 査 票

ご出産おめでとうございます。ご出産から今までの間にどのようにお感じになったかを
お知らせください。今日だけでなく、過去7日間にあなたが感じられたことに最も近い
答えにアンダーラインを引いてください。必ず10項目に答えてください。

例） 幸せだと感じた。　　　はい、常にそうだった
　　　　　　　　　　　　　はい、たいていそうだった
　　　　　　　　　　　　　いいえ、あまり度々ではなかった
　　　　　　　　　　　　　いいえ、全くそうではなかった

"はい、たいていそうだった"と答えた場合は過去7日間のことをいいます。この様な
方法で質問にお答えください。

〔質問〕

1.　笑うことができたし、物事のおかしい面もわかった。

　　　　　　　　　　いつもと同様にできた
　　　　　　　　　　あまりできなかった
　　　　　　　　　　明らかにできなかった
　　　　　　　　　　全くできなかった

2.　物事を楽しみにして待った。

　　　　　　　　　　いつもと同様にできた
　　　　　　　　　　あまりできなかった
　　　　　　　　　　明らかにできなかった
　　　　　　　　　　ほとんどできなかった

3.　物事が悪くいった時、自分を不必要に責めた。

　　　　　　　　　　はい、たいていそうだった
　　　　　　　　　　はい、時々そうだった
　　　　　　　　　　いいえ、あまり度々ではない
　　　　　　　　　　いいえ、そうではなかった

4.　はっきりした理由もないのに不安になったり、心配した。

　　　　　　　　　　いいえ、そうではなかった
　　　　　　　　　　ほとんどそうではなかった
　　　　　　　　　　はい、時々あった
　　　　　　　　　　はい、しょちゅうあった

5. はっきりした理由もないのに恐怖に襲われた。

> はい、しょちゅうあった
> はい、時々あった
> いいえ、めったになかった
> いいえ全くなかった

6. することがたくさんあって大変だった。

> はい、たいてい対処できなかった
> はい、いつものようにはうまく対処しなかった
> いいえ、たいていうまく対処した
> いいえ、普段通りに対処した

7. 不幸せなので、眠りにくかった。

> はい、ほとんどいつもそうだった
> はい、ときどきそうだった
> いいえ、あまり度々ではなかった
> いいえ、全くなかった

8. 悲しくなったり、惨めになった。

> はい、たいていそうだった
> はい、かなりしばしばそうだった
> いいえ、あまり度々ではなかった
> いいえ、全くそうではなかった

9. 不幸せなので、泣けてきた

> はい、たいていそうだった
> はい、かなりしばしばそうだった
> ほんの時々あった
> いいえ、全くそうではなかった

10. 自分自身を傷つけるという考えが浮かんできた。

> はい、かなりしばしばそうだった
> 時々そうだった
> めったになかった
> 全くなかった

Maltese

Kwestjonarja Dwar L-emmozzjonijiet wara it-tqala

Kif qeghda thossok? Nixtiequ nkunu nafu kif qeghda thossok. Jekk joghgbok immarka wahda li thoss li tghodd fil kas tieghek, ta' kif hassejtek f'dawn l-ahhar sebghat ijiem, u mhux kif qeghda thossok illum. Hawn taht hawn ezempju diga lest.

Jiena hassejtni ferhana
    Iva, il hinn kollu
    <u>Iva, hafna drabi</u>
    Le, mhux ta' spiss
    Le, qatt
Din tfisser li "jien hassejtni ferhana hafna drabi" f'din l-ahhar gimgha

Jekk joghgbok ghamel id-domandi l-ohrajn bl-istess mod.

FL-AHHAR SEBGHAT IJIEM

1. Kont kapaci nifrah u nhares lejn is-sabih tal-hajja
    Bhas soltu
    Mhux daqs is-soltu
    Zgur li mhux bhas soltu
    Zgur li le

2. Kien jkolli certu hegga ghal dak li jkun sejr naghmel
    Bhas soltu
    Aktarx inqas mis-soltu
    Zgur li nqas mis-soltu
    Ftit li xejn

3. Tajt tort lili nnifsi ghal xejn b'xejn meta l-affarijiet marru hazing
    Kwazi dejjem
    Iva, kultant
    Mhux ta' spiss
    Le, qatt

4. Hassejtni nervuza u nkwietata ghal xejn b'xejn
    Le, lanqas xejn
    Rari hafna
    Iva, kultant
    Iva, spiss

5. Hassejtnis bezghana u qabadni paniku anke ghal xejn b'xejn
    Iva, hafna drabi
    Iva kultanta
    Le, mhux spiss
    Le, qatt

6. Ma stajt inlahhaq ma xejn
    Iva, hafna drabi hassejtni li ma stajtx inlahhaq
    Iva, kultant hassejtni li ma kontx kapaci nlahhaq bhas-soltu
    Le, hafna drabi stajt nlahhaq
    Le, lahhaqt bhas-soltu

7. Tant kemm hasejtni mdejqa li kont insibha bi tqila biex norqod
    Kwazi dejjem
    Iva, kultant
    Mhux ta' spiss
    Le, qatt

8. Hassejtni mdejqa u misserabli
    Iva, kwazi l-hinn kollu
    Iva ta' spiss
    Le, mhux ta' spiss
    Le, qatt

9. Tant hassejtni mdejqa li minn daqqiet kien itini l-biki
    Iva, kwazi l-hinn kollu
    Iva, ta' spiss
    Xi kultant
    Le, qatt

10. Kienu jiguni xi hsibijiet li naghmel hsara lili nnifsi
    Iva, ta' spiss
    Xi, kultant
    Rari, hafna
    Qatt

Norwegian

1. Har du siste 7 dager kunnet le og se det komiske i en situasjon?
   Like mye som vanlig
   Ikke riktig så mye som jeg pleier
   Klart mindre enn jeg pleier
   Ikke i det hele tatt

2. Har du siste 7 dager gledet deg til ting som skulle skje?
   Like mye som vanlig
   Noe mindre enn jeg pleier
   Klart mindre enn jeg pleier
   Nesten ikke i det hele tatt

3. Har du siste 7 dager bebreidet deg selv uten grunn når noe gikk galt?
   Ja, nesten hele tiden
   Ja, av og til
   Ikke særlig ofte
   Nei, aldri

4. Har du siste 7 dager vært nervøs eller bekymret uten grunn?
   Nei, slett ikke
   Nesten aldri
   Ja, iblant
   Ja, veldig ofte

5. Har du siste 7 dager vært redd eller fått panikk uten grunn?
   Ja, svært ofte
   Ja, noen ganger
   Sjelden
   Nei, aldri

6. Har du siste 7 dager følt at det har blitt for mye for deg?
   Ja, jeg har stort sett ikke fungert i det hele tatt
   Ja, iblant har jeg ikke klart å fungere som jeg pleier
   Nei, for det meste har jeg klart meg bra
   Nei, jeg har klart meg like bra som vanlig

7. Har du siste 7 dager vært så ulykkelig at du har hatt vanskeligheter med å sove?
> Ja, for det meste
> Ja, iblant
> Ikke særlig ofte
> Nei, ikke i det hele tatt

8. Har du siste 7 dager felt deg nedfor eller ulykkelig?
> Ja, det meste av tiden
> Ja, ganske ofte
> Ikke særlig ofte
> Nei, ikke i det hele tatt

9. Har du siste 7 dager vært så ulykkelig at du har grått?
> Ja, nesten hele tiden
> Ja, veldig ofte
> Ja, det har skjedd iblant
> Nei, aldri

10. Har tanken på å skade deg selv streifet deg, de siste 7 dagene?
> Ja, nokså ofte
> Ja, av og til
> Ja, såvidt
> Aldri

Translated by Malin Eberhard-Gran

Portuguese

Como teve recentemente um bebé, gostariamos de saber como se sente. Por favor, sublinhe a resposta que melhor indique o modo como se sente *desde há 7 dias* e não apenas hoje.

Aqui está um exemplo:

Senti-me feliz:
   Sim, sempre
   <u>Sim, quase sempre</u>
   Näo, poucas vezes
   Näo, nunca

Isto quereria dizer: "Senti-me feliz quase sempre durante os últimos sete dias". Por favor, complete as outras questöes do mesmo modo.

DESDE HÁ 7 DIAS

1. Tenho sido capaz de me rir e ver o lado-divertido das coisas
   Tanto como dantes
   Menos do que antes
   Muito menos do que antes
   Nunca

2. Tenho tido esperança no futuro
   Tanta como sempre tive
   Bastante menos do que costumava ter
   Muito menos do que costumava ter
   Quase nenhuma

3. Tenho-me culpado sem necessidade quando as coisas correm mal
   Sim, a maioria das vezes
   Sim, algumas vezes
   Raramente
   Näo, nunca

4. Tenho estado ansiosa ou preocupada sem motivo
   Näo, Nunca
   Quase nunca
   Sim, por vezes
   Sim, muitas vezes

5. Tenho-me sentido com medo, ou muito assustada, sem grande motivo
   Sim, muitas vezes
   Sim, por vezes
   Não, raramente
   Não, nunca

6. Tenho sentido que são coisas demais para mim
   Sim, a maioria das vezes não tenho conseguido resolvê-las
   Sim, por vezes não tenho conseguido resolvê-las como dantes
   Não, a maioria das vezes resolvo-as fácilmente
   Não, resolvo-as tão bem como dantes

7. Tenho-me sentido tão infeliz que durmo mal
   Sim, quase sempre
   Sim, por vezes
   Raramente
   Não, nunca

8. Tenho-me sentido triste ou muito infeliz
   Sim, quase sempre
   Sim, muitas vezes
   Raramente
   Não, nunca

9. Tenho-me sentido tão infeliz que choro
   Sim, quase sempre
   Sim, muitas vezes
   Só, às vezes
   Não, nunca

10. Tive ideias de fazer mal a mim mesma
    Sim, muitas vezes
    Por vezes
    Muito raramente
    Nunca

Punjabi

Kujh din pahilan tuhada bachha paeda hoiaa hae aatae eh jananna chahudae han ke tuseen kis taran maehsoos karde ho. Pishlae ik haphtae ton jis yaran vee tuseen maehsoos kita cee oos barae mehar-bani karke dhhuck veen khanae vich nishan laga-dioo.

Eh ik aapdea layee namoona tiar kita hoiaa hae (e.g.)

Maen khush rahee cee
> Bahut vaar
> <u>Kayee vaar</u>
> Bahut vaar nahin
> Bilkul nahin

Aaseen nishan swal de dujae hissea wich laeeyah hae.

Pishlae sat dina vich

1. Meree hasnae khadnae dee isha cee
    Pehilan jinee hee
    Agae nalon ghat
    Kadae kadae
    Bil-kul nahin

2. Maen dilhon khushee de nal cam karna chohundee cee
    Peilan wang hee
    Agae nalon kujh ghat
    Bil-kul agae nalon ghat
    Kadae vee nahin

3. Maen binan kisae karan aapnae aapda kasoor samajh-dee cee
    Bahut var
    Kayee var
    Bahut var nahin
    Bil-kul nahin

4. Maen bina kisae khash karan hee chinta phikar kardee cee
    Kadae vee nahin
    Bahut hee ghat
    Kadae kadae
    Bahut var

5. Maen bina kisae khash karan toen hee dar atae ghabrahat mahaesoos kardee cee
    Bahut var
    Kadee kadae
    Bahut var nahin
    Bil-kul nahin

6. Maen innee udas cee ke maen kisae tarah de tangee jan fikar valee gall sahar nahin sakdee cee
    Bahut var
    Kayee var
    Pehilan nalon kujh ghat
    Agae wang hee

7. Maenu gaman de dukh nal neend nahin aaundee cee
    Bahut var
    Kadae kadae
    Bahut var nahin
    Bil-kul nahin

8. Maen udas rahindee cee
    Bahut var
    Kayee var
    Bahut var nahin
    Bil-kul nahin

9. Maen innee udas cee kae maen rondee rahindee cee
    Bahut var
    Kayee var
    Kadae kadae
    Bil-kul nahin

10. Mera dil karda cee kae maen aapnae aap noon kujh kar lavan
    Buhat var
    Kadae kadae
    Bahut var nahin
    Bil-kul nahin

Translated by Asha Day

Slovenian

Ker ste pred kratkim rodili dojenčka, bi radi izvedeli, kako se počutite. Prosim, PODČRTAJTE odgovor, ki približno opisuje Vaše počutje V ZADNJIH 7 DNEH, in ne le Vašega počutja danes.

1. Uspe mi, da se nasmejim in vidim smešno plat stvari:

   ○ tako, kot mi je to vedno uspelo,
   ○ manj kot prej,
   ○ veliko manj kot prej,
   ○ sploh ne.

2. Veselim se stvari:

   ○ tako, kot sem se vedno,
   ○ manj kot prej,
   ○ precej manj kot prej,
   ○ skoraj ne.

3. Po nepotrebnem se obremenjujem, kadar gredo stvari narobe:

   ○ večino časa,
   ○ nekaj časa,
   ○ redko,
   ○ nikoli.

4. Brez pravega razloga sem tesnobna in zaskrbljena:

   ○ sploh ne,
   ○ komaj kdaj,
   ○ včasih,
   ○ zelo pogosto.

5. Brez pravega razloga se počutim prestrašeno ali panično:

   ○ pogosto,
   ○ včasih,
   ○ redko,
   ○ sploh ne.

6. Stvari se mi nakopičijo:

   ○ večino časa jih ne zmorem obvladati,
   ○ včasih jih ne obvladam tako dobro kot prej,
   ○ večino časa jih precej dobro obvladujem,
   ○ obvladujem jih tako dobro kot vedno.

7. Bila sem tako nesrečna, da sem slabo spala:

   ◦ večino časa,
   ◦ včasih,
   ◦ redko,
   ◦ sploh ne.

8. Počutila sem se žalostno ali nesrečno:

   ◦ večino časa,
   ◦ precej pogosto,
   ◦ redko,
   ◦ sploh ne.

9. Bila sem tako nesrečna, da sem jokala:

   ◦ večino časa,
   ◦ precej pogosto,
   ◦ občasno,
   ◦ nikoli.

10. Pomislila sem, da bi si kaj naredila:

   ◦ precej pogosto,
   ◦ včasih,
   ◦ skoraj nikoli,
   ◦ nikoli.

Spanish

SUS SENTIMIENTOS DURANTE LA SEMANA PASADA

1. He podido reír y ver el lado bueno de las cosas:
   Tanto como siempre
   No tanto ahora
   Mucho menos
   No, no he podido

2. He mirado al futuro con placer:
   Tanto como siempre
   Algo menos de lo que solía hacer
   Definitivamente menos
   No, nada

3. Me he culpado innecesariamente cuando las cosas marchaban mal:
   Sí, la mayor parte de las veces
   Sí, algunas veces
   No muy a menudo
   No, nunca

4. He estado ansiosa y preocupada sin motivo:
   No, nada
   Casi nada
   Sí, a veces
   Sí, a menudo

5. He sentido miedo y pánico sin motivo alguno:
   Sí, bastante
   Sí, a veces
   No, no mucho
   No, nada

6. Las cosas me superaban, me sobrepasaban:
   Sí, la mayor parte de las veces
   Sí, a veces
   No, casi nunca
   No, nada

7. Me ha sentido tan infeliz, que he tenido dificultad para dormir:
   Sí, casi siempre
   Sí, a veces
   No muy a menudo
   No, nada

8. Me he sentido triste y desgraciada:
   Sí, casi siempre
   Sí, bastante a menudo
   No muy a menudo
   No, nada

9. He sido tan infeliz que he estado llorando:
   Sí, casi siempre
   Sí, bastante a menudo
   Sólo ocasionalmente
   No, nunca

10. He pensado en hacerme daño a mí misma:
    Sí, bastante a menudo
    A veces
    Casi nunca
    No, nunca

Swedish

Eftersom Du nyligen fått barn, skulle vi vilja veta hur Du mår. Var snäll och stryk under det svar, som bäst stämmer överens med hur Du känt Dig under de sista 7 dagarna, inte bara hur Du mår idag.

Här är ett exempel, som redan är ifyllt:

Jag har känt mig lycklig:
Ja, hela tiden
Ja, för det mesta
Nej, inte särskilt ofta
Nej, inte alls

Detta betyder: Jag har känt mig lycklig mest hela tiden under veckan som har gått. Var snäll och fyll i de andra frågorna på samma sätt:

UNDER DE SENASTE 7 DAGARNA

1. Jag har kunnat se tillvaron från den ljusa sidan:
Lika bra som vanligt
Nästan lika bra som vanligt
Mycket mindre än vanligt
Inte alls

2. Jag har glatt mig åt saker som skall hända:
Lika mycket som vanligt
Något mindre än vanligt
Mycket mindre än vanligt
Inte alls

3. Jag har lagt skulden på mig själv onödigt mycket när något har gått snett:
Ja, för det mesta
Ja, ibland
Nej, inte så ofta
Nej, aldrig

4. Jag har känt mig rädd och orolig utan egentlig anledning:
Nej, inte alls
Nej, knappast alls
Ja, ibland
Ja, mycket ofta

5. Jag har känt mig strämd eller panikslagen utan speciell anledning:
   Ja, mycket ofta
   Ja, ibland
   Nej, ganska sällan
   Nej, inte alls

6. Det har kört ihop sig för mig och blivit för mycket:
   Ja, mesta tiden har jag inte kunnat ta itu med något alls
   Ja, ibland har jag inte kunnat ta itu med saker lika bra som vanligt
   Nej, för det mesta har jag kunnat ta itu med saker ganska bra
   Nej, jag har kunnat ta itu med saker precis som vanligt

7. Jag har känt mig så ledsen och olycklig att jar har haft svårt att sova:
   Ja, mesta tiden
   Ja, ibland
   Nej, sällan
   Nej, aldrig

8. Jag har känt mig ledsen och nere:
   Ja, för det mesta
   Ja, rätt ofta
   Nej, sällan
   Nej, aldrig

9. Jag har känt mig så olycklig att jag har gråtit:
   Ja, nästan jämt
   Ja, ganska ofta
   Bara någon gång
   Aldrig

10. Tankar på att göra mig själv illa har förekommit:
    Ja, rätt så ofta
    Ja, ganska ofta
    Ja, då och då
    Aldrig

Urdu

آپ کیسی ہیں؟

جیسا کہ آپ کا حال ہی الحمد پہلے ہی پرائے ۔ اب آپ کیسا محسوس کر رہی ہیں؟۔

مہربانی سے اپنے جواب (جو قریباً آپ کے حالات کے حالیان نیں) کے نیچے لائن لگائیں کہ پچھلے سات دن سے آپ کی طبیعت کیسی ہے؟ ۔ نہ صرف کہ آج کیسا محسوس کر رہی ہیں ۔

یہ مثال کے طور پر ہند سوال ہیں ۔ جو آپ کے مکمل کیے اٹھائیے جائیں ۔ آپ ایسی دیکھ کر اسی طرح اپنے جواب بنائیں ۔ یعنی اس جواب کے نیچے لائن لگائیں جو آپ کی حالات کے زیادہ قریب ہے ۔

میں نے اپنے آپ کو خوش محسوس کیا ہے ۔

اکثر اوقات ۔

کبھی کبھی دقت ۔

نہیں اکثر نہیں ۔

نہیں بالکل نہیں ۔

" اس کا مطلب ہوا کہ پچھلے سننے کے دوران اپنے آپ کو کبھی کبھی دقت خوش محسوس کیا ہے "

مہربانی سے دوسرے سوالوں کے جواب بھی اسی طرح دیں ۔

پچھلے سات دنوں سے

1. چیزوں کے مزاحیہ رخ کی طرف دیکھ کر میں ہنسی ۔
   جیسا میں پہلے کرتی تھی ۔
   اب کے اتنا نہیں ہنسی ۔
   یقیناً اب کے اتنا نہیں ہنسی جتنا پہلے ہنستی تھی ۔
   بالکل نہیں ۔

2. میں چیزوں کے واقع ہونے کا خوشی سے انتظار کرتی ہوں ۔ میں چیزوں کی پرواہ کرتی ہوں ۔
   اتنا ہی جتنا پہلے کرتی تھی ۔
   پہلے سے ذرا کم ۔
   یقیناً اس کے ذرا کم جتنا پہلے کرتی تھی ۔
   بالکل نہیں ذرا بھی پرواہ نہیں کرتی ۔

3. جب کوئی چیز غلط ہو گئی ۔ تو میں نے اپنے آپ کو قصور دار مانا ۔ بغیر وجہ کے اپنے آپ کو
   الگ مقام پر رکھیے ؟

پچھلے سات دنوں سے (جاری ہے)

اکثر ایسا کرتی ہوں ۔
کبھی کبھار ایسا کرتی ہوں ۔
میں اکثر اپنے آپ کو مجرم نہیں کہتی ۔
بالکل نہیں اپنے کو الزام نہیں دیتا ۔

4. میں نے اپنے آپ کو پریشان اور بغیر خاص وجہ کے مکر مند محسوس کیا ہے ۔ !
بالکل یہیں ۔
شاید کبھی ۔ ؟
ہاں کبھی کبھار ۔ ؟
اکثر اوقات

5. میں نے آپ کو فسردہ اور گھبرا یا بُرا محسوس کیا ہے !
ہاں بہت زیادہ ۔ ؟
کبھی کبھار ۔
زیادہ یہیں ۔
بالکل یہیں ۔

6. چیزیں میرے سر پر سوار رہی ہیں ؟
ہاں اکثر اوقات یہیں کہ چیزوں کو بالکل یہیں نمٹا سکی ۔
ہاں میں کبھی کبھی چیزوں کو اس طرح یہیں نمٹا سکی جیسے پہلے ۔
ہیں اکثر میں چیزوں کو اچھی طرح یہیں کر سکی ۔
یہیں میں بالکل مثبت سے کوئی کام پورا نہ کر سکی ۔

7. میں اتنی ناخوشی تھی کہ مجھے اچھی طرح سونے میں مشکل پیش آئی ۔
بہت دفعہ ایسا ہوا ۔
کبھی کبھار ایسا ہوا ۔
کبھی ایسا اکثر یہیں سوتا ۔
ایسا بالکل یہیں ہوتا کہ میں سو نہ سکوں ۔

8. میں نے اپنے آپ کو بہت تھکیلیں اور بُرا طرح محسوس کیا ۔
اکثر اوقات ۔
ہاں اکثر ایسا ہوا ۔
یہیں اکثر یہیں کبھی کبھار ۔
یہیں بالکل یہیں ۔

9. میں اتنی ناخوشی ہو لی کہ میں روتی رہی ۔
ہاں اکثر ایسا ہوا ۔
جی اکثر اوقات ایسا ہوا ۔
صرف کبھی کبھار ایسا ہوا ۔
بالکل یہیں ۔ ناخوشی تھی مگر رونی یہیں ۔

10. اپنے آپ پر بریست کفتہ آیا اور اپنے آپ کو ماؤنے کو جی چاہا ۔
اکثر ایسا ہوا ۔ ایسا کبھی کبھار ہوا ۔
شاید ہی کبھی ایسا خیال آیا آیا ہے ۔
یہیں ایسا بالکل یہیں محسوس کیا ۔

Vietnamese

Vì chị vừa sanh cháu bé nên chúng tôi muốn biết chị cảm thấy thế nào. Xin hãy gạch dích câu trả lời phù hợp nhất với cảm giác của chị trong 7 ngày qua. Không phải chỉ hôm nay mà thôi.

Sau dây là một thí dụ:
Chị có cảm thấy vui vẻ không ?

 _ Vâng, luôn luôn lúc nào cũng vậy.
 _ <u>Vâng, hầu như lúc nào cũng vậy.</u>
 _ Không, không thường lắm.
 _ Không, không bao giờ.

Câu trả lời trên có nghĩa là : Ề Tôi hầu như lúc nào cũng cảm thấy vui vẻ Ề trong suốt tuần qua. Xin hãy hoàn tất những câu hỏi dưới đây theo cách chỉ dẫn trên.

TRONG 7 ngày qua

1. Chị có thể tức cười và thấy được phần hài hước của những chuyện khôi hài không ?
    Vẫn như trước.
    Ít hơn.
    Chắc chắn là ít hơn.
    Không bao giờ.

2. Chị có nhìn vào tương lai với niềm hân hoan/vui vẻ không ?
    Vẫn như trước.
    Ít hơn trước.
    Chắc chắn là ít hơn trước.
    Gần như không có.

3. Chị có tự đổ lỗi cho chính mình một cách quá đáng khi chuyện xãy ra không được như ý không ?
    Rất thường xuyên.
    Thỉnh thoảng.
    Rất hiếm.
    Không bao giờ.

4. Chị có cảm thấy không yên tâm hay lo sợ một cách vô lý không ?
    Không bao giờ.
    Rất hiếm.
    Thỉnh thoảng.
    Rất thường xuyên.

5. Chị có cảm thấy sợ sệt hay hoảng hốt một cách vô lý không ?
   Vâng, nhiều lắm.
   Vâng, đôi khi.
   Không, rất hiếm.
   Không khi nào.

6. Chị có cảm thấy mọi việc xảy ra đều quá sức chịu đựng của chị hay không ?
   Tôi luôn luôn cảm thấy quá sức chịu đựng.
   Chỉ thỉnh thoảng.
   Hầu như lúc nào tôi cũng cảm thấy thoải mái.
   Tôi luôn luôn cảm thấy thoải mái.

7. Chị có cảm giác buồn đến mức khó ngủ không ?
   Vâng, hầu như lúc nào cũng vậy.
   Vâng, thỉnh thoảng.
   Không thường lắm.
   Không khi nào.

8. Chị có cảm thấy buồn hay khổ sở không ?
   Vâng, hầu như lúc náo cũng vậy.
   Vâng, rất thường.
   Không thường lắm.
   Không khi nào.

9. Chị có quá u buồn đến độ thường hay khóc không ?
   Vâng, hầu như lúc nào cũng vậy.
   Vâng, rất thường.
   Không, không thường lắm.
   Không khi nào.

10. Chị có bao giờ có ý nghĩ tự tử không.
    Vâng, rất thường.
    Đôi khi.
    Rất ít khi.
    Không khi nào.   Xin cám ơn chị.

References

Adams, C. (2002) The EPDS: Guidelines for its use as part of a maternal mood assessment. *Community Practitioner*, **75**, 394–395.

Aitken, P. & Jacobson, R. (1997) Knowledge of the Edinburgh Postnatal Depression Scale among psychiatrists and general practitioners. *Psychiatric Bulletin*, **21**, 550–552.

American Psychiatric Association (1980) *Diagnostic and Statistical Manual of Mental Disorders* (3rd edn) (DSM–III). Washington, DC: APA.

—— (1994) *Diagnostic and Statistical Manual of Mental Disorders* (4th edn) (DSM–IV). Washington, DC: APA.

Ancill, R., Hilton, S., Carr, T. *et al* (1986) Screening for antenatal and postnatal depressive symptoms in general practice using a microcomputer-delivered questionnaire. *Journal of the Royal College of General Practitioners*, **36**, 276–279.

Angeli, N. & Grahame, K. (1990) Screening for postnatal depression. *Midwife, Health Visitor and Community Nurse*, **26**, 428–430.

Appleby, L. (1991) Suicide during pregnancy and in the first postnatal year. *BMJ*, **302**, 137–140.

——, Gregoire, A., Platz, C., *et al* (1994) Screening women for high risk of postnatal depression. *Journal of Psychosomatic Research*, **38**, 539–545.

——, Warner, R., Whitton, A., *et al* (1997) A controlled study of fluoxetine and cognitive–behavioural counselling in the treatment of postnatal depression. *BMJ*, **314**, 932–936.

Areias, M. E., Kumar, R., Barros, H., *et al* (1996a) Comparative incidence of depression in women and men, during pregnancy and after childbirth. Validation of the Edinburgh Postnatal Depression Scale in Portuguese mothers. *British Journal of Psychiatry*, **169**, 30–35.

——, ——, ——, *et al* (1996b) Correlates of postnatal depression in mothers and fathers. *British Journal of Psychiatry*, **169**, 36–41.

Atkinson, K. A. & Rickel, A. U. (1984) Postpartum depression in primiparous parents. *Journal of Abnormal Psychology*, **93**, 115–119.

Bågedahl-Strindlund, M. & Monsen Borjesson, K. (1998) Postnatal depression: a hidden illness. *Acta Psychiatrica Scandinavica*, **98**, 272–275.

Ballard, C. G., Davis, R., Cullen, P. C., *et al* (1994) Prevalence of postnatal psychiatric morbidity in mothers and fathers. *British Journal of Psychiatry*, **164**, 782–788.

Barclay, L. & Kent, D. (1998) Recent immigration and the misery of motherhood: a discussion of pertinent issues. *Midwifery*, **14**, 4–9.

Barker, W. (1998) Let's trust our instincts. *Community Practitioner*, **71**, 305.

Barnett, B., Lockhart, K., Bernard, D., *et al* (1993) Mood disorders among mothers of infants admitted to a mothercraft hospital. *Journal of Paediatric and Child Health*, **29**, 270–275.

——, Matthey, S. & Boyce, P. (1999) Migration and motherhood: a response to Barclay & Kent (1998). *Midwifery*, **15**, 203–207.

Beck, C. T. & Gable, R. K. (2001) Comparative analysis of the performance of the Postpartum Depression Screening Scale with two other depression instruments. *Nursing Research*, **50**, 242–250.

Beck, A. T., Ward, C. H., Mendelsohn, M., et al (1961) An inventory for measuring depression. *Archives of General Psychiatry*, **4**, 53–63.

Bedford, A. & Foulds, G. (1978) *Delusions, Symptoms, States. State of Anxiety and Depression (Manual)*. Windsor: National Foundation for Educational Research.

Benvenuti, P., Ferrara, M., Niccolai, C., et al (1999) The Edinburgh Postnatal Depression Scale: validation for an Italian sample. *Journal of Affective Disorders*, **53**, 137–141.

Bergant, A. M., Nguyen, T., Heim, K., et al (1998) Deutschsprachige Fassung und Validierung der 'Edinburgh postnatal depression scale' [German language version and validation of the Edinburgh postnatal depression scale]. *Deutsche Medizinische Wochenschrift*, **123**, 35–40.

Boath, E. & Henshaw, C. (2001) The treatment of postnatal depression: a comprehensive literature review. *Journal of Reproductive and Infant Psychology*, **19**, 215–248.

—, Cox J., Lewis, M., et al (1999) When the cradle falls: the treatment of postnatal depression in a psychiatric day hospital compared with routine primary care. *Journal of Affective Disorders*, **53**, 143–151.

Boyce, P. M., Stubbs, J. & Todd, A. L. (1993) The Edinburgh Postnatal Depression Scale: validation for an Australian sample. *Australian and New Zealand Journal of Psychiatry*, **27**, 472–476.

Brockington, I. (1996) *Motherhood and Mental Health*, pp. 234–244. Oxford: Oxford University Press.

Brugha, T. S., Sharp, H. M., Cooper, S. A., et al (1998) The Leicester 500 Project. Social support and the development of postnatal depressive symptoms: a prospective cohort survey. *Psychological Medicine*, **28**, 63–79.

—, Wheatley, S., Taub, N. A., et al (2000) Pragmatised randomised trial of antenatal intervention to prevent postnatal depression by reducing psychosocial risk factors. *Psychological Medicine*, **30**, 1273–1281.

Buist, A. E., Barrnett, B. E. W., Milgrom, J., et al (2002) To screen or not to screen – that is the question in perinatal depression. *Medical Journal of Australia*, **177** (suppl.), S101–S105.

Campbell, S. B. & Cohn, J. F. (1997) The timing and chronicity of postpartum depression: implications for infant development. In *Postpartum Depression and Child Development* (eds L. Murray & P. J. Cooper), pp. 165–201. New York: Guilford Press.

Carpiniello, B., Pariante, C. M., Serri, F., et al (1997) Validation of the Edinburgh Postnatal Depression Scale in Italy. *Journal of Psychosomatic Obstetrics and Gynaecology*, **18**, 280–285.

Clark, G. (2000) Discussing emotional health in pregnancy: the Edinburgh Postnatal Depression Scale. British Journal of Community Nursing, 5, 91–98.

Clifford, C., Day, A. & Cox, J. (1997) Women's health after birth. Developing the use of the EPDS in a Punjabi-speaking community. British Journal of Midwifery, 5, 616–619.

—, —, —, et al (1999) A cross-cultural analysis of the use of the EPDS in health visiting practice. *Journal of Advanced Nursing*, **30**, 655–664.

Cogill, S. R., Caplan, H. L., Alexandra, H., et al (1986) Impact of maternal postnatal depression on cognitive development of young children. BMJ, **292**, 1165–1167.

Comport, M. (1990) *Surviving Motherhood*. Bath: Ashgrove Press.

Condon, J. T. & Corkindale, C. J. (1997) The assessment of depression in the postnatal period: a comparison of four self-report questionnaires. *Australian and New Zealand Journal of Psychiatry*, **31**, 353–359.

Cooper, P. J. & Murray, L. (1995) Course and recurrence of postnatal depression. Evidence for the specificity of the diagnostic concept. *British Journal of Psychiatry*, **166**, 191–195.

— & — (1997) The impact of psychological treatments of postpartum depression on maternal mood and infant development. In *Postpartum Depression and Child Development* (eds L. Murray & P. Cooper), pp. 202–221. New York: Guilford Press.

—, —, Hooper, R., *et al* (1996) The development and validation of a predictive index for postpartum depression. *Psychological Medicine*, **26**, 627–634.

—, Tomlinson, M., Swartz, L., *et al* (1999) Post-partum depression and the mother–infant relationship in a South African peri-urban settlement. *British Journal of Psychiatry*, **175**, 554–558.

Corney, R. H. (1980) Health visitors and social workers. *Health Visitor*, **53**, 409–413.

Cox, J. L. (1983) Postnatal depression: a comparison of Scottish and African women. *Social Psychiatry*, **18**, 25–28.

— (1986) *Postnatal Depression: A Guide for Health Professionals*. Edinburgh: Churchill Livingstone.

— (1988) The life event of childbirth: sociocultural aspects of postnatal depression. In *Motherhood and Mental Illness* (vol. 2.) (eds R. Kumar & I. Brockington), pp. 64–75. London: John Wright.

— (1989) Postnatal depression: a serious and neglected postpartum complication. *Baillière's Clinical Obstetrics and Gynaecology*, **3**, 839–855.

— (1996) Perinatal mental disorder – a cultural approach. *International Review of Psychiatry*, **8**, 9–16.

— (1998) Patients as parents: possible impact of changing childbirth and faltering families. *Archives of Women's Mental Health*, **1**, 55–61.

— (1999) Perinatal mood disorders in a changing culture. A transcultural European and African perspective. *International Review of Psychiatry*, **11**, 103–110.

— & Holden, J. (eds) (1994) *Perinatal Psychiatry: Use and Misuse of the Edinburgh Postnatal Depression Scale*. London: Gaskell.

—, Connor, Y. & Kendell, R. E. (1982) Prospective study of the psychiatric disorders of childbirth. *British Journal of Psychiatry*, **140**, 111–117.

—, Rooney, A., Thomas, P. F., *et al* (1984) How accurately do mothers recall postnatal depression? Further data from a 3-year follow-up study. *Journal of Psychosomatic Obstetrics and Gynaecology*, **3**, 185–189.

—, Holden, J. M. & Sagovsky, R. (1987) Detection of postnatal depression. Development of the 10-item Edinburgh Postnatal Depression Scale. *British Journal of Psychiatry*, **150**, 782–786.

—, Gerrard, J. & Cookson, D. (1993) Development and audit of Charles Street Parent and Baby Day Unit, Stoke-on-Trent. *Psychiatric Bulletin*, **17**, 711–713.

—, Chapman, G., Murray, D., *et al* (1996) Validation of the Edinburgh Postnatal Depression Scale (EPDS) in non-postnatal women. *Journal of Affective Disorders*, **39**, 185–189.

Coyle, B. & Adams, C. (2002) The EPDS: guidelines for its use as part of maternal mood assessment. *Community Practitioner*, **75**, 394–395.

Coyle, N., Jones, I., Robertson, E., *et al* (2000) Variation at the serotonin transporter gene influences susceptibility to bipolar affective puerperal psychosis. *Lancet*, **366**, 1490–1491.

Cryan, E., Keogh, F., Connolly, E., *et al* (2001) Depression among postnatal women in an urban Irish community. *Irish Journal of Psychological Medicine*, **18**, 5–10.

Cullinan, R. (1991) Health visitor intervention in postnatal depression. *Health Visitor*, **64**, 412–414.

Da-Silva, V. A., Moraes-Santos, A. R., Carvalho, M. S., *et al* (1998) Prenatal and postnatal depression among low income Brazilian women. *Brazilian Journal of Medical and Biological Research*, **31**, 799–804.

Derogatis, L. R. & Cleary, P. A. (1977) Confirmation of the dimensional structure of SCL-90: a study in construct validation. *Journal of Clinical Psychiatry*, **33**, 981–989.

Dragonas, T., Golding, J., Ignatyeva, R., *et al* (eds) (1996) *Pregancy in the Nineties. The European Longitudinal Study of Pregnancy and Childhood*. Bristol: Sansom.

Eastwood, P. (1995) Promoting peer group support with postnatally depressed women. *Health Visitor*, **68**, 148–150.

Eberhard-Gran, M., Eskild, A., Tambs, K., *et al* (2001) The Edinburgh Postnatal Depression Scale: validation in a Norwegian community sample. *Nordic Journal of Psychiatry*, **55**, 113–117.

Edhborg, M., Lundh, W., Seimyr, L, *et al* (2001) The long-term impact of postnatal depressed mood on mother–child interaction: a preliminary study. *Journal of Reproductive and Infant Psychology*, **19**, 61–71.

Elliott, S. A. (1994) Uses and misuses of the Edinburgh Postnatal Depression Scale in primary care: a comparison of models developed in health visiting. In *Perinatal Psychiatry. Use and Misuse of the Edinburgh Postnatal Depression Scale* (eds J. Cox & J. Holden), pp. 221–232. London: Gaskell.

— & Leverton, T. J. (2000) Is the EPDS a magic wand? 'Myths' and the evidence base. *Journal of Reproductive and Infant Psychology*, **18**, 296–307.

—, Sanjack, M. & Leverton, T. (1988) Parents groups in pregnancy: a preventive intervention for postnatal depression? In *Marshaling Social Support. Formats, Processes and Effects* (ed. B. H. Gottlieb), pp. 87–110. London, Sage Publications.

—, Leverton, T. J., Sanjack, M., *et al* (2000) Promoting mental health after childbirth: a controlled trial of primary prevention of postnatal depression. *British Journal of Clinical Psychology*, **39**, 223–241.

—, Gerrard, J., Ashton, C., *et al* (2001) Training health visitors to reduce levels of depression after childbirth: an evaluation. *Journal of Mental Health*, **10**, 613–625.

Evans, J., Heron, J., Francomb, H., *et al* (2001) Cohort study of depressed mood during pregnancy and after childbirth. *BMJ*, **323**, 257–260.

Evins, G. G., Theofrastous, J. P. & Galvin, S. L. (2000) Postpartum depression: a comparison of screening and routine clinical evaluation. *American Journal of Obstetrics and Gynecology*, **182**, 1080–1082.

Felice, E. (1998) *Emotional Disorders during Pregnancy and the Postnatal Period: A Prospective Study of Maltese Women*. MPhil Thesis. Keele: Keele University.

Fisch, R. Z., Tadmor, O. P., Dankner, R. (1997) Postnatal depression: a prospective study of its prevalence, incidence and psychosocial determinants in an Israeli sample. *Journal of Obstetrics and Gynaecology Research*, **23**, 547–554.

Fitzgerald, M. H., Ing, M., Ya, T. H., *et al* (1988) *Hear Our Voices: Trauma, Birthing and Mental Health among Cambodian Women*. Sydney: Transcultural Mental Health Centre, Paramatta.

Flaherty, J. A., Gaviria, F. M., Pathak, D., *et al* (1988) Developing instruments for cross-cultural psychiatric research. *Journal of Nervous and Mental Disease*, **176**, 257–263.

Freeling, P. (1992) Implications for general practice training and education. In *The Prevention of Depression and Anxiety: The Role of the Primary Care Team* (eds R. Jenkins, J. Newton & R. Young), pp. 57–68. London: HMSO.

Gair, S. (1999) Distress and depression in new motherhood: research with adoptive mothers highlights important contributing factors. *Child and Family Social Work*, **4**, 55–66.

Georgiopoulos, A. M., Bryan, T. L., Wollan, P., *et al* (2001) Routine screening for postpartum depression. *Journal of Family Practice*, **50**, 117–122.

Gerrard, J., Holden, J. M., Elliott, S. A., *et al* (1994) A trainer's perspective of an innovative training programme to teach health visitors about the detection, treatment and prevention of postnatal depression. *Journal of Advanced Nursing*, **18**, 1825–1832.

Ghubash, R., Abou-Saleh, M. T. & Daradkeh, T. K. (1997) The validity of the Arabic Edinburgh Postnatal Depression Scale. *Social Psychiatry and Psychiatric Epidemiology*, **32**, 474–476.

Gilbody, S. M., House, A. O. & Sheldon, T. A. (2001) Routinely administered questionnaires for depression and anxiety: a systematic review. *BMJ*, **332**, 406–409.

Glasser, S. & Barell, V. (1999) Depression scale for research in and identification of postpartum depression [in Hebrew]. *Harefuah*, **136**, 764–768.

Glaze, R. & Cox, J. L. (1991) Validation of a computerised version of the 10-item (self-rating) Edinburgh Postnatal Depression Scale. *Journal of Affective Disorders*, **22**, 73–77.

Goldberg, D. P. (1972) *The Detection of Psychiatric Illness by Questionnaires*. Oxford: Oxford University Press.

—— (1992) Early diagnosis and secondary prevention. In *Prevention of Depression and Anxiety in General Practice: The Role of the Practice Team* (eds R. Jenkins, J. Newton & R. Young), pp. 33–39. London, HMSO.

——, Cooper, B., Eastwood, M. R., *et al* (1970) A standardised psychiatric interview for use in community surveys. *British Journal of Preventive Social Medicine*, **24**, 1–23.

Gordan, R. E. & Gordan, K. K. (1960) Social factors in prevention of postpartum emotional adjustment. *Obstetrics and Gynecology*, **15**, 433–438.

Gotlib, I. H., Whiffen, V. E., Mount, J. H., *et al* (1989) Prevalence rates and demographic characteristics associated with depression in pregnancy and the postpartum. *Journal of Consulting and Clinical Psychology*, **57**, 269–274.

Green, J. M. (1998) Postnatal depression or perinatal dysphoria? Findings from a longitudinal community-based study using the Edinburgh Postnatal Depression Scale. *Journal of Reproductive and Infant Psychology*, **16**, 143–155.

—— & Murray, D. (1994) The use of the Edinburgh Postnatal Depression Scale in research to explore the relationship between antenatal and postnatal dysphoria. In *Perinatal Psychiatry. Use and Misuse of the Edinburgh Postnatal Depression Scale* (eds J. Cox & J. Holden), pp. 180–198. London: Gaskell.

——, Coupland, V. A. & Kitzinger, J. V. (1990) Expectations, experiences and psychological outcomes of childbirth: a prospective study of 825 women. *Birth*, **17**, 15–24.

Griepsma, J., Marcollo, J., Casby, C., *et al* (1994) The incidence of postnatal depression in a rural area and the needs of affected women. *Australian Journal of Advanced Nursing*, **11**, 19–23.

Guedeney, N. & Fermanian, J. (1998) Validation study of the French version of the Edinburgh Postnatal Depression Scale (EPDS). New results about use and psychometric properties. *European Psychiatry*, **13**, 83–89.

——, ——, Guelfi, J. D., *et al* (2000) The Edinburgh Postnatal Depression Scale (EPDS) and the detection of major depressive disorders in early postpartum: some concerns about false negatives. *Journal of Affective Disorders*, **61**, 107–112.

Hamilton, M. (1960) A rating scale for depression. *Journal of Neurology, Neurosurgery and Psychiatry*, **23**, 56–62.

Harris, B., Huckle, P., Thomas, R., *et al* (1989) The use of rating scales to identify post-natal depression. *British Journal of Psychiatry*, **154**, 813–817.

Harrison, M. (1992) Linking with voluntary and community resources: Homestart consultancy. In *Prevention of Depression and Anxiety in General Practice: The Role of the Practice Team* (eds J. Jenkins, R. Newton & R. Young), pp. 140–144. London: HMSO.

Hay, D. F., Pawlby, S., Sharp, D., *et al* (2001) Intellectual problems shown by 11-year-old children whose mothers had postnatal depression. *Journal of Child Psychology and Psychiatry*, **42**, 871–889.

Hearn, G., Iliff, A., Jones, I., *et al* (1998) Postnatal depression in the community. *British Journal of General Practice*, **48**, 1064–1066.

Heh, S. S. (2001) Validation of the Chinese version of the Edinburgh Postnatal Depression Scale: detecting postnatal depression in Taiwanese women. *Nursing Research (China)*, **9**, 105–113.

Henshaw, C. A. (2000) *A Longitudinal Study of Postnatal Dysphoria* (MD thesis). Aberdeen: University of Aberdeen.

Holden, J. M. (1986) Counselling for health visitors. In *Postnatal Depression – A Guide for Health Professionals* (ed. J. L. Cox), pp. 53–57. Edinburgh: Churchill Livingstone.

— (1988) *A Randomised Controlled Trial of Counselling by Health Visitors in the Treatment of Postnatal Depression.* MPhil thesis. Edinburgh: University of Edinburgh.

— (1990) Emotional problems associated with childbirth. In *Midwifery Practice: Postnatal Care* (eds J. Alexander, V. Levy & S. Roch), pp. 45–61. Basingstoke: Macmillan.

— (1991) Postnatal depression: its nature, effects, and identification using the Edinburgh Postnatal Depression Scale. *Birth*, **18**, 211–221.

— (1994a) Using the Edinburgh Postnatal Depression Scale in clinical practice. In *Perinatal Psychiatry. Use and Misuse of the Edinburgh Postnatal Depression Scale* (eds J. Cox & J. Holden), pp. 125–144. London: Gaskell.

— (1994b) Can non-psychoitic depression be prevented? In *Perinatal Psychiatry. Use and Misuse of the Edinburgh Postnatal Depression Scale* (eds J. Cox & J. Holden), pp. 54–81. London: Gaskell.

— (1996) The role of health visitors in postnatal depression. *International Review of Psychiatry*, **8**, 79–86.

—, Sagovsky, R. S. & Cox, J. L. (1989) Counselling in a general practice setting: a controlled study of health visitor intervention in the treatment of postnatal depression. *BMJ*, **298**, 223–226.

Holt, W. J. (1995) The detection of postnatal depression in general practice using the Edinburgh Postnatal Depression Scale. *New Zealand Medical Journal*, **108**, 57–59.

Jadresic, E. & Araya, R. (1995) Prevalence of postpartum depression and associated factors in Santiago, Chile [Spanish]. *Revista Medica de Chile*, **123**, 694–699.

—, Jara, C., Miranda, M., *et al* (1992) Tastornos emocionales en el embarazo y el peuerperio: estudio prospective de 108 mujeres [Emotional disorders in pregnancy and the puerperium: a prospective study of 108 women]. *Revista Chilena de Neuro-Psiquiatria*, **30**, 99–106.

—, Araya, R. & Jara, C. (1995) Validation of the Edinburgh Postnatal Depression Scale (EPDS) in Chilean postpartum women. *Journal of Psychosomatic Obstetrics and Gynaecology*, **16**, 187–191.

Johnstone, S. J., Boyce, P. M., Hickey, A. R., *et al* (2001) Obstetric risk factors for postnatal depression in urban and rural community samples. *Australian and New Zealand Journal of Psychiatry*, **35**, 69–74.

Josefsson, A., Berg, G., Nordin, C., *et al* (2001) Prevalence of depressive symptoms in late pregnancy and postpartum. *Acta Obstetricia et Gynecologica Scandinavica*, **80**, 251–255.

Kaplan, P. S., Bachorowski, J. & Zarlengo-Strouse, P. (1999) Child-directed speech produced by mothers with symptoms of depression fails to promote associative learning in 4-month old infants. *Child Development*, **70**, 560–570.

Katzenelson, S. K., Maizel, S., Zilber, N., *et al* (2000) Validation of the Hebrew version of the Edinburgh Postnatal Depression Scale: methods, results and application [abstract in Hebrew]. In *Abstracts of the Tenth Congress of the Israel Psychiatric Association, Jerusalem, April 2000* [in Hebrew], p. 163. Tel Aviv: Israel Psychiatric Association.

Kendell, R. E., Rennie, D., Clarke, J. A., *et al* (1981) The social and obstetric correlates of psychiatric admission in the puerperium. *Psychological Medicine*, **11**, 341–350.

—, Chalmers, J. C. & Platz, C. (1987) Epidemiology of puerperal psychoses. *British Journal of Psychiatry*, **150**, 662–673.

Kit, L. K., Janet, G. & Jegasothy, R. (1997) Incidence of postnatal depression in Malaysian women. *Journal of Obstetrics and Gynaecology Research*, **23**, 85–89.

Kumar, R. (1994) Postnatal mental illness: a transcultural perspective. *Social Psychiatry and Psychiatric Epidemiology*, **29**, 250–264.

Laungani, P. (2000) Postnatal depression across cultures: conceptual and methodological considerations. *International Journal of Health Promotion and Education*, **38**, 86–94.

Lawrie, T. A., Hofmeyr, G. J., De Jager, M., *et al* (1998) Validation of the Edinburgh Postnatal Depression Scale on a cohort of South African women. *South African Medical Journal*, **88**, 1340–1344.

Lee, D. T., Yip, S. K., Chiu, H. F., *et al* (1998) Detecting postnatal depression in Chinese women. Validation of the Chinese version of the Edinburgh Postnatal Depression Scale. *British Journal of Psychiatry*, **172**, 433–437.

Leviston, A. & Downs, M. (1999) Open space. When instinct is not enough. *Community Practitioner*, **72**, 184–185.

Lewinsohn, P. M., Antonuccio, D. O., Steinmetz, J. L., *et al* (1984) *The Coping with Depression Course: A Psycho-Educational Intervention for Unipolar Depression*. Eugene, OR: Castalsa.

Lloyd-Williams, M., Friedman, T. & Rudd, N. (2000) Criterion validation of the Edinburgh Postnatal Depression Scale as a screening tool for depression in patients with advanced metastatic cancer. *Journal of Pain and Symptom Management*, **20**, 259–265.

Lundh, W. & Gyllang, C. (1993) Use of the Edinburgh Postnatal Depression Scale in some Swedish child health care centres. *Scandinavian Journal of Caring Sciences*, **7**, 149–154.

Lussier, V., David, H., Saucier, J.-F., *et al* (1996) Self-rating assessment of postnatal depression: a comparison of the Beck Depression Inventory and the Edinburgh Postnatal Depression Scale. *Pre- and Peri-Natal Psychology Journal*, **11**, 81–91.

MacArthur, C., Winter, H. R., Bick, D. E., *et al* (2002) Effects of redesigned community postnatal care on women's health 4 months after birth: a cluster randomised controlled trial. *Lancet*, **359**, 378–385.

Malan, D. H., Heath, E. S., Bacal, H. A., *et al* (1975) Psychodynamic changes in untreated neurotic patients – II. Apparently genuine improvements. *Archives of General Psychiatry*, **32**, 110–126.

Marks, M. N. & Kumar, R. (1993) Infanticide in England and Wales. *Medical Science and Law*, **33**, 329–339.

Matthey, S. (2003) Calculating clinically significant change in postnatal depression studies using the Edinburgh Postnatal Depression Scale. *Journal of Affective Disorders*, in press.

—, Barnett, B. E. & Elliott, A. (1997) Vietnamese and Arabic women's responses to the Diagnostic Interview Schedule (depression) and self-report questionnaires: cause for concern. *Australian and New Zealand Journal of Psychiatry*, **31**, 360–369.

—, Barnett, B. E., Kavanagh, D. J., *et al* (2001) Validation of the Edinburgh Postnatal Depression Scale for men, and comparison of item endorsement with their partners. *Journal of Affective Disorders*, **64**, 175–184.

McNair, D. M. & Lorr, M. (1964) An analysis of mood in neurotics. *Journal of Abnormal and Social Psychology*, **69**, 620–627.

Mead, N., Bower, P. & Gask, L. (1997) Emotional problems in primary care: what is the potential for increasing the role of nurses? *Journal of Advanced Nursing*, **26**, 879–890.

Milgrom, J., Martin, P. R. & Negri, L. M. (1999) *Treating Postnatal Depression*. Chichester: John Wiley & Sons.

Minde, K., Tidmarsh, L. & Hughes, S. (2001) Nurses' and physicians' assessment of mother–infant mental health at the first postnatal visits. *Journal of the American Academy of Child and Adolescent Psychiatry*, **40**, 803–810.

Misri, S., Kostaras, X., Fox, D., *et al* (2000) The impact of partner support in the treatment of postpartum depression. *Canadian Journal of Psychiatry. Revue Canadienne de Psychiatrie*, **45**, 554–558.

Morgan, M., Matthey, S., Barnett, B., *et al* (1997) A group programme for postnatally distressed women and their partners. *Journal of Advanced Nursing*, **26**, 913–920.

Morrell, C. J., Spiby, H., Stewart, P., *et al* (2000) Costs and benefits of community postnatal support workers: a randomised controlled trial. *Health Technology Assessment*, **4**, 1–100.

117

Murray, D. & Cox, J. L. (1990) Identifying depression during pregnancy with the Edinburgh Postnatal Depression Scale (EPDS). *Journal of Reproductive and Infant Psychology*, **8**, 99–107.

—, —, Chapman, G., *et al* (1995) Childbirth: life event or start of a long-term difficulty? Further data from the Stoke-on-Trent controlled study of postnatal depression. *British Journal of Psychiatry*, **166**, 595–600.

Murray L. (1988) Effects of postnatal depression on infant development. The contribution of direct studies of early mother–infant interactions. In *Motherhood and Mental Illness* (vol. 2) (eds R. Kumar & I. F. Brockington), pp. 159–191. London: John Wright.

— & Carothers, A. D. (1990) The validation of the Edinburgh Post-Natal Depression Scale on a community sample. *British Journal of Psychiatry*, **157**, 288–290.

—, Fiori-Cowley, A., Hooper, R., *et al* (1996*a*) The impact of postnatal depression and associated adversity on early mother–infant interactions and later infant outcome. *Child Development*, **67**, 2512–2526.

—, Hipwell, A., Hooper, R., *et al* (1996*b*) The cognitive development of 5-year-old children of postnatally depressed mothers. *Journal of Child Psychology and Psychiatry and Allied Disciplines*, **37**, 927–935.

—, Cooper, P. J., Wilson, A., *et al* (2003) Controlled trial of the short- and long-term effect of psychological treatment of post-partum depression. 2: Impact on the mother–child relationship and child outcome. *British Journal of Psychiatry*, **182**, 420–427.

Muzik, M., Klier, C. M., Rosenblum, K. L., *et al* (2000) Are commonly used self-report inventories suitable for screening postpartum depression and anxiety disorders? *Acta Psychiatrica Scandinavica*, **102**, 71–73.

Nhiwatiwa, S., Patel, V. & Acuda, W. (1988) Predicting postnatal mental disorders with a screening questionnaire: a prospective cohort study. *Journal of Epidemiological Health*, **52**, 262–266.

Nielsen Forman, D., Videbech, P., Hedegaard, M., *et al* (2000) Postpartum depression: identification of women at risk. *British Journal of Obstetrics and Gynaecology*, **107**, 1210–1217.

Oakley, A. (1980) *Women Confined: Towards a Sociology of Childbirth*. Oxford: Martin Robertson.

Oates, M. (1989) Management of major mental illness in pregnancy and the puerperium. *Baillière's Clinical Obstetrics and Gynaecology*, **3**, 905–921.

— (1996) Psychiatric services for women following childbirth. *International Review of Psychiatry*, **8**, 87–98.

— (2001) Deaths from psychiatric causes. In *Why Mothers Die 1997–1999. The Confidential Enquiries into Maternal Deaths in the United Kingdom* (ed. G. Lewis), pp. 65–187. London: Royal College of Gynaecologists and Obstetricians.

—, Cox, J. L., Neema, S., *et al* (2003) Postnatal depression across countries and cultures: a qualitative study. *British Journal of Psychiatry*, in press.

O'Hara, M. W. (1994) Postpartum depression: identification and measurement in a cross-cultural context. In *Perinatal Psychiatry. Use and Misuse of the Edinburgh Postnatal Depression Scale* (eds J. Cox & J. Holden), pp. 145–168. London: Gaskell.

— (1995) *Postpartum Depression: Causes and Consequences*. New York: Springer.

—, Zakoski, E. M., Philipps, L. H., *et al* (1990) Controlled prospective study of postpartum mood disorders: comparison of childbearing and nonchildbearing women. *Journal of Abnormal Psychology*, **99**, 3–15.

—, Stuart, S., Gorman, L., *et al* (2000) Efficiency of interpersonal psychotherapy for postpartum depression. *Archives of General Psychiatry*, **57**, 1039–1045.

Okano, T., Murata, M., Masuji, F., *et al* (1996) Validation and reliability of a Japanese version of the EPDS. *Archives of Psychiatric Diagnosis and Clinical Evaluation*, **7**, 525–533.

—, Nagata, S., Hasegawa, M., *et al* (1998) Effectiveness of antenatal education about postnatal depression: a comparison of two groups of Japanese mothers. *Journal of Mental Health (UK)*, **7**, 191–198.

Olioff, M. (1991) The application of cognitive therapy to postnatal depression. In *The Challenge of Cognitive Therapy: Applications to Non-Traditional Populations* (eds T. M. Vallis, J. L. Howes & P. C. Miller), pp. 111–133. New York: Plenum Press.

Onozawa, K., Glover, V., Adams, D., *et al* (2001) Infant massage improves mother–infant interaction for mothers with postnatal depression. *Journal of Affective Disorders*, **63**, 201–207.

Ormel, H., Koester, M., Van Der Brink, W., *et al* (1990) The extent of non-recognition of mental problems in primary care and its effect on management and outcome. In *The Public Health Impact of Mental Disorder* (eds D. Goldberg & D. Tantum). Bern: Hogrefe and Huber.

Pace, C. (1992) A health education library in general practice. In *The Prevention of Depression and Anxiety: The Role of the Primary Care Team* (eds R. Jenkins, J. Newton & R. Young), pp. 131–135. London, HMSO.

Painter, A. (1995) Health visitor identification of postnatal depression. *Health Visitor*, **68**, 138–140.

Patel, V., DeSouza, N. & Rodrigues, M. (2003) Postnatal depression and infant growth and development in low income countries: a cohort study from Goa, India. *Archives of Disease in Childhood*, **88**, 34–37.

Pitt, B. (1968) 'Atypical' depression following childbirth. *British Journal of Psychiatry*, **114**, 1325–1335.

Pitts, F. (1995) Group work 1. Comrades in adversity: the group approach. *Health Visitor*, **68**, 144–145.

Pop, V. J., Komproe, I. H. & Van Somm, M. J. (1992) Characteristics of the Edinburgh Postnatal Depression Scale in the Netherlands. *Journal of Affective Disorders*, **26**, 105–110.

Radloff, L. S (1977) The CES–D Scale: a self-report depression scale for research in the general population. *Applied Psychological Measures*, **1**, 385–401.

Roy, A., Gang, P., Cole, K., et al (1993) Use of Edinburgh Postnatal Depression Scale in a North American population. *Progress in Neuro-Psychopharmacology and Biological Psychiatry*, **17**, 501–504.

Royal College of Psychiatrists (2000) *Perinatal Maternal Mental Health Services* (Council Report CR88). London: Royal College of Psychiatrists.

Schaper, A. M, Rooney, B. L., Kay, N. R., *et al* (1994) Use of the Edinburgh Postnatal Depression Scale to identify postpartum depression in a clinical setting. *Journal of Reproductive Medicine*, **39**, 620–624.

Scottish Intercollegiate Guidelines Network (2002) *Postnatal Depression and Puerperal Psychosis: a National Clinical Guideline*. Edinburgh: Scottish Intercollegiate Guidelines Network.

Seeley, S. (2001) Postnatal depression and maternal mental health: a public health priority. *CPHVA Conference Proceedings, October 2001*, pp. 16–19. London: CPHV.

—, Murray, L. & Cooper, P. J. (1996) Postnatal depression: the outcome for mothers and babies of health visitor intervention. *Health Visitor*, **69**, 135–138.

Shakespeare, J. (2002) Health visitor screening for PND using the EPDS: a process study. *Community Practitioner*, **5**, 381–384.

Sharp, D., Hay, D. F., Pawlby, S., *et al* (1995) The impact of postnatal development on boys' intellectual development. *Journal of Child Psychology and Psychiatry*, **36**, 1315–1336.

Shereshefsky, P. M. & Lockman, R. F. (1973) Comparison of counselled and non-counselled groups. In *Psychological Aspects of a First Pregnancy and Early Postnatal Adaptation* (eds P. M. Shereshefsky & U. Yarrow), pp. 151–163. New York: Raven Press.

Sinclair, D. & Murray, L. (1998) Effects of postnatal depression on children's adjustment to school. Teacher's reports. *British Journal of Psychiatry*, **172**, 58–63.

Small, R., Johnston, V. & Orr, A. (1997) Depression after childbirth: the views of medical students and women compared. *Birth*, **24**, 109–115.

—, Lumley, J., Donohue, L., *et al* (2000) Randomised controlled trial of midwife led debriefing to reduce maternal depression after operative childbirth. *BMJ*, **321**, 1043–1047.

Snaith, R. P. (1983) Pregnancy-related psychiatric disorder. *British Journal of Hospital Medicine*, **29**, 450–456.

Spinelli, M. G. (1997) Interpersonal psychotherapy for depressed antepartum women: a pilot study. *American Journal of Psychiatry*, **154**, 1028–1030.

Spitzer, R. L., Endicott, J. & Robins, E. (1978) Research Diagnostic Criteria Instrument no. 58. *Archives of General Psychiatry*, **35**, 273–282.

Stamp, G. E. & Crowther, C. A. (1994) Postnatal depression: a South Australian prospective study. *Australian and New Zealand Journal of Obstetrics and Gynaecology*, **34**, 164–167.

—, Williams, A. S. & Crowther, C. A. (1995) Evaluation of antenatal and postnatal support to overcome postnatal depression: a randomized, controlled trial. *Birth*, **22**, 138–143.

Stein, A., Gath, D. H., Bucher, J., *et al* (1991) The relationship between postnatal depression and mother–child interaction. *British Journal of Psychiatry*, **158**, 46–52.

Stein, G. (1998) Postpartum and related disorders. In *General Adult Psychiatry* (vol. 2) (eds G. Stein & G. Wilkinson), pp. 903–953. London: Gaskell.

Steinberg, S. I. & Bellavance, F. (1999) Characteristics and treatment of women with antenatal and postpartum depression. *International Journal of Psychiatry in Medicine*, **29**, 209–233.

Stern, G. & Kruckman, I. (1983) Multi-disciplinasry perspectives on postpartum depression: an anthropological critique. *Social Science and Medicine*, **17**, 1027–1041.

Stuart, S., Couser, G., Schilder, K., *et al* (1998) Post-partum anxiety and depression: onset and comorbidity in a community sample. *Journal of Nervous and Mental Disease*, **186**, 420–424.

Sundelin, C. & Håkansson, A. (2000) The importance of the Child Health Services to the health of children. Summary of the state-of-the-art document from the Sigtuna conference on Child Health Services with a view to the future. *Acta Paediatrica Supplementum*, **434**, 76–79.

Suzuki, H. (2001) Evolution of the perinatal care system. *Pediatrics International*, **43**, 194–196.

Tamaki, R., Murata, M. & Okano, T. (1997) Risk factors for postpartum depression in Japan. *Psychiatry and Clinical Neuroscience*, **51**, 93–98.

Taylor, E. (1989) Postnatal depression: what can a health visitor do? *Journal of Advanced Nursing*, **14**, 877–886.

Taylor, S. (1998) Instinct or knowledge? *Community Practitioner*, **71**, 427.

Tcixeira, J. M. A., Fisk, N. M. & Glover, V. (1999) Association between maternal anxiety in pregnancy and increased uterine artery resistance index: cohort based study. *BMJ*, **318**, 153–157.

Thome, M. (1991) Emotional distress during the postpartum period from the second to the sixth month, assessed by community nurses. *Nordic Midwifery Research (Oslo)*, **9**, 25–27.

— (1992) Mat heilsugæsluhjúkrunarfræðinga á vanlíðan íslenskra kvenna 2–6 mánuðum eftir barnsburð. *Hjúkrun*, **68**, 8–15.

— (1996) *Distress in Mothers with Difficult Infants in the Community. An Intervention Study*. Doctoral dissertation. Edinburgh: Queen Mary College, Edinburgh, & Open University.

— (1999) Geðheilsuvernd Mæðra Eftir Fæðingu. Greining á vanlíðan með Edinborgar-þunglyndiskvarðanum og viðtölum. Rannsóknarstofnun í hjúkrunarfræði og Háskólaútgáfan.

— & Alder, B. (1999) A telephone intervention to reduce fatigue and symptom distress in mothers with difficult infants in the community. *Journal of Advanced Nursing*, **29**, 128–137.

Thompson, W. M., Harris, B., Lazarus, J., et al (1998) A comparison of the performance of rating scales used in the diagnosis of postnatal depression. *Acta Psychiatrica Scandinavica*, **98**, 224–227.

Thorpe, K. (1993) A study of the use of the Edinburgh Postnatal Depression Scale with parent groups outside the postpartum period. *Journal of Reproductive and Infant Psychology*, **11**, 119–125.

—, Dragonas, T. & Golding, J. (1992) The effects of psychological factors on the mother's emotional well-being during early parenthood: a cross-cultural study of Britain and Greece. *Journal of Reproductive and Infant Psychology*, **10**, 191–248.

Tully, C., Watson, C. & Abrams, A. (1998) Postnatal depression: training health visitors to use the EPDS. *Community Practitioner*, **71**, 213–215.

Vega-Dienstmaier, J. M., Suarez, G. M. & Sanchez, M. C. (2002) Validation of a Spanish version of the Edinburgh Postnatal Depression Scale. *Actas Espanolas de Psiquiatria*, **30**, 106–111.

Warner, R., Appleby, L., Whitton, A., et al (1997) Attitudes toward motherhood in postnatal depression: development of the Maternal Attitudes Questionnaire. *Journal of Psychosomatic Research*, **43**, 351–358.

Watson, J. P., Elliott, S. A., Rugg, A. J., et al (1984) Psychiatric disorder in pregnancy and the first postnatal year. *British Journal of Psychiatry*, **144**, 453–462.

Webster, M. L., Thompson, J. M., Mitchell, E. A., et al (1994) Postnatal depression in a community cohort. *Australian and New Zealand Journal of Psychiatry*, **28**, 42–49.

—, Linnane, J. W., Dibley, L. M., et al (2000) Improving antenatal recognition of women at risk for postnatal depression. *Australian and New Zealand Journal of Obstetrics and Gynaecology*, **40**, 409–412.

Welburn, V. (1980) *Postnatal Depression*. Glasgow: Collins.

Wickberg, B. & Hwang, C. P. (1996a) Counselling of postnatal depression: a controlled study on a population-based Swedish sample. *Journal of Affective Disorders*, **39**, 209–216.

— & — (1996b) The Edinburgh Postnatal Depression Scale: validation on a Swedish community sample. *Acta Psychiatrica Scandinavica*, **94**, 181–184.

— & — (1997) Screening for postnatal depression in a population-based Swedish sample. *Acta Psychiatrica Scandinavica*, **95**, 62–66.

Wieck, A., Kumar, R., Hirst, A. D, et al (1991) Increased sensitivity of dopamine receptors and recurrence of affective psychosis after childbirth. *BMJ*, **303**, 613–616.

Williams, P., Tarnopolsky, A. & Hand, D. (1980) Case definition and case identification in psychiatric epidemiology. *Psychological Medicine*, **10**, 101–114.

Wisner, K. L, James, M. P. & Findling, R. L. (1996) Antidepressant treatment during breast-feeding. *American Journal of Psychiatry*, **153**, 1132–1137.

World Health Organization (1992) *The ICD–10 Classification of Mental and Behavioural Disorders*. Geneva: WHO.

— (1999) *World Health Report, 1999: Making a Difference*. Geneva: World Health Organization.

Wrate, R. M., Rooney, A. C., Thomas, P. F., et al (1985) Postnatal depression and child development. A three-year follow-up study. *British Journal of Psychiatry*, **146**, 622–627.

Yonkers, K. & Little, B. (eds) (2001) *Management of Psychiatric Disorders in Pregnancy*. London: Arnold.

Yoshida, K., Yamashita, H., Ueda, M., *et al* (2001) Postnatal depression in Japanese mothers and the reconsideration of 'Satogaeri bunben'. *Pediatrics International*, **43**, 189–193.

Zelkowitz, P. & Milet, T. H. (1995) Screening for postpartum depression in a community sample. *Canadian Journal of Psychiatry*, **40**, 80–86.

— & — (1996) Postpartum psychiatric disorders: their relationship to psychological adjustment and marital satisfaction in the spouses. *Journal of Abnormal Psychology*, **105**, 281–285.

Zigmond, A. S. & Snaith, R. P. (1983) The Hospital Anxiety and Depression Scale. *Acta Psychiatrica Scandinavica*, **67**, 361–370.

Zung, W. W. K. (1965) A self-rating depression scale. *Archives of General Psychiatry*, **12**, 63–70.

Index